birds and ghosts

jess richards

¶

Published by Linen Press, London 2023
8 Maltings Lodge
Corney Reach Way
London W4 2TT
www.linen-press.com

Cover design: Jess Richards
Typeset by Zebedee
Printed by Lightning Source
ISBN: 978-1-7391777-0-6

About the Author

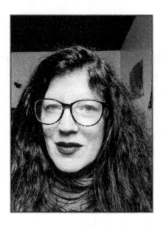

Jess Richards was born in Wales and raised in Scotland. She is the author of three literary fiction novels: Costa shortlisted *Snake Ropes*, *Cooking with Bones* and *City of Circles* (Sceptre). She also writes creative nonfiction, vispo, short fiction and poetry which have been published in various anthologies. Her fine art / creative writing PhD project, Illusions, Transformations, and Iterations; storytelling as fiction, image, and artefact, earned her a place on the Dean's List at Massey University, Aotearoa New Zealand. *Birds and Ghosts* is a book-length work of creative nonfiction written when New Zealand borders were closed due to Covid-19. In October 2022 Jess, her wife, and two stripy cats returned to live in the UK. They now live in Yorkshire where Jess works at the University of Leeds.

Praise for Birds and Ghosts

"Grief needs space all around it, and air to breathe through." This lucent, transcendent book is both a meditation on grief, loneliness, love, disconnection and connection, and a journey into the uniquely sensitive, often visceral, nuanced imagination of an extraordinarily attuned narrator. The reader enters the writer's waking dreams, where the borders of perception dissolve and where prose and poetry intertwine. Jess Richards's inner life is her superpower.
– Catherine Smith, poet and fiction writer

It's a myth we were ever alive, and *Birds and Ghosts* dazzles through figurations of that myth. If you've ever been grief-struck with love, split from a founding sense of home, pierced by our strange human institutions, and healed in relations with other-than-human beings – including the gift that is language – this memoir of transition years will feel like a truth-telling. "A ragged bird goes to a golden cage and burns like a phoenix." Loneliness keeps Jess Richards company; pouring through this book, that loneliness looks like love.
– Lisa Samuels, author of *Symphony for Human Transport* and *Breach*

In this stunning book, Jess Richards creates a new vocabulary for loneliness, loss, and desire. Brilliantly interweaving image and text, prose and poetry, she threads together stories of breakup, death, and new love. Releasing the haunting presence of the past, this book sets stories in motion, the imagination in flight, and words on fire.
– Jacob Edmond, author of *Make It the Same: Poetry in the Age of Global Media*

This is an astounding piece of writing. Part poetry, part prose, but all a storyteller at the height of their craft pulling you into their beautiful, tender, and often heart-breaking world.
– Kerry Hudson, author of *Lowborn*

This fearless and beautiful book is as luminous as it is haunting. *Birds and Ghosts* blurs and transcends the borders between life and death, poetry and prose, drawing and language. Tracing the arc of grief, Richards reveals how loss opens us into a deeper truth of love.
– Diane Comer, author of *The Braided River: Migration and the Personal Essay*

At once tender and unnerving, gentle and brutal. *Birds and Ghosts* is one of those books that opens a new pathway to the heart and clears an unused route to the mind.
– Gigi Fenster, author of *Feverish* and *A Good Winter*

In *Birds and Ghosts*, acclaimed novelist Jess Richards lets the masks of fiction slip to tenderly trace the teardrop paths of her own fugue and fugitive states: bereavement, loneliness, heartbreak, migration, pandemic, supernatural experiences, a late diagnosis of autism. Caught up in a perfect storm of grief and revelation, words and memories whirl into distinctive, fluid forms: prose poems, illustrations, fables, neologisms, hauntings, odes to the writer's wife, elegies for baby blackbirds, skein in and out of silence in the pages of this searching and innovative memoir. As a profound meditation on death, *Birds and Ghosts* contains passages so beautiful and wise one might read them to a terminally ill friend or family member. As a personal tribute to a beloved father, the book honours an artist and teacher who nourished his daughter's exceptional imagination, without ever knowing that the sensitivity they shared might have had another, clinical, name. In lyrical, synaesthetic, often painfully perceptive reflections, like and yet unlike Anand Prahlad and Joanne Limburg, Richards reaches for, and draws near, the unique, ungraspable nature of self-on-the-spectrum. Exploring universal experiences, challenging stereotypes, and expressing the writer's truths in a murmuration of language all her own, *Birds and Ghosts* offers sky-bridges of empathy and understanding to neurotypical and neurodiverse readers alike. An act of generous vulnerability, deep insight, and consummate artistry, Jess Richards's autobiography makes a compelling contribution to the rapidly growing fields of autistic and neuroqueer literature – and deserves, too, a prominent place in the broader landscapes of life writing and experimental prose.
– Naomi Foyle, poet, essayist and SF novelist

Author's note—

This book is a creative nonfiction narrative which was written in 2021. While it is based on my recollection of events, names and identities have been changed or are composites.

How do you grieve for him, when you can't visit his grave?
I grieve in the language of birds and ghosts.

The Language of Birds and Ghosts

There's a nest growing in the back garden. It's eight feet above the ground, half-hidden on a wooden frame tangled with grapevines and climbing roses. For days, a pair of blackbirds have been weaving, expanding their nest with twigs, leaves, strips of plastic.

Seen through thickening rose leaves, the nest has solid sides but the base is full of holes. Small eggs would fall, smash. Break open and spill. What would spill out? The early stages of tiny dark feathers, the edge of a claw, a partly-grown skull? Blackbird chicks are naked and blind when they first hatch. I've seen photographs of them online. Half-nightmare, half-beak.

Curled on the sofa with my wife, Morgan, we watch a nature documentary. She leans against me and I stroke her silvery shoulder-length hair.

Baby blackbirds are made of hunger.

Open, close. Open, close.

Two weeks later, the adult blackbirds haven't been around for a while. Morgan hasn't seen them going to the nest either, though she's noticed them flitting in and out of the garden. We consider the idea they build many nests in different places and choose the best one.

> *The best nest must:*
> *be out of reach of cats,*
> *be made from strong materials,*
> *not have holes*
> *never sway during gales.*
> *The best nest must:*
> *be out of reach of humans.*

> *If a human enters your nest, death visits.*

In our street the back gardens are narrow and I doubt the blackbirds notice the thin fences which separate one set of humans from another.

Though the nest seems empty, I don't get too close in case it isn't. There are a lot of things I don't do. I don't climb up and check for an invisible bird who's sitting on invisible eggs. I don't clap my hands at the neighbour's cats when they're stalking something I can't see. I don't push a broom up there, to topple the nest so I can see what materials it's made from.

I want to hold the empty nest in my hands and examine how it's constructed. I want to take their house into our home and cradle it. Birds are master-weavers, collectors, and thieves. They have carefully selected every piece of nesting material. Their eyes will have darted, fixed on something. A perfectly curved twig. A soft texture. Strength? Colour? The beak will have gripped, pincer-tight.

Though I don't touch the empty nest in case it's bad luck, I keep wondering why the blackbirds have built a nest they aren't using. Perhaps they decided not to breed and add more blackbirds into an already overcrowded garden. After all, the world must seem unpredictable and dangerous to them as well right now. In Wellington, urban roads are quiet. The sky is empty of aeroplanes and often full of chattering squawking shrieking birds. And like me, blackbirds don't really belong in New Zealand.

But this is where we are.

Sometimes the sound of an unfamiliar shrieking bird wakes me at night and I go outside to listen, in case it's the sound of grotesque chicks learning to scream. With blue eyes gleaming, Morgan says the sound might be owls. But at night-time, I often think about blackbirds.

Tonight, I've got period cramps and can't sleep. Morgan keeps telling me I'll love the menopause just like she did—that it's brilliant when periods finally end. I've not heard anyone else say that before, but then again, Morgan often has an unusual take on things. At three in the morning after finding no easy answer on google as to whether or not my menopause will happen any time soon, I look up blackbirds again.

The screenlight from my phone shines my hands pale. The images of their chicks are miniature monsters, ghouls, spirits. The full-grown birds seem softer and their thin necks look far more breakable.

The wind is raging and it's dark outside. My mum calls me on Skype. She's at home in Scotland, bathed in white daylight. Her image is unstable and her henna hair shines orange. Behind her are the tall windows of my childhood home with bird-silhouette stickers on the panes to stop birds flying into the glass.

She sounds tearful. 'You would have been visiting right now. Bloody corvid.'

'I know,' I reply. Covid does sound similar to the name for the crow family and I don't want to be annoying and correct her. 'We'll visit as soon as it's safe to travel, to fly.'

'But when will that be?' Her mouth gapes strangely and she covers it with a pixelated hand.

'I don't know.'

Looking over her shoulder at the stickers of birds, I remember other times I've spent in that room. Before it was a lived-in space, it was derelict for many years. When I was a teenager, my friends used to come round and we'd spend hours in there without adults.

I search for her eyes behind the reflection of the screen in her glasses as I ask, 'What have you been doing with yourself?'

'Ooh, I haven't shown you.' Her chair scrapes on the wooden floor, she lurches into close view and then disappears. Her voice gets fainter as she calls, 'Talk amongst yourself.'

On the screen the white sky blurs around the windows. I imagine my dad appearing faintly on this screen as a ghost-man, or flying up to the windows as a bird, tapping his beak on the pane.

Talking to me in bird-tap-code, telling me he only pretended to die.

The white-sky-windows blur my eyes and my mum's footfall returns. Her strengthening voice says, 'Look—I've been making leaves. Then I'll make a vine to bind them all together. It'll be a scarf. I've got a pattern.'

A vague shape of green, bronze, purple fills the screen. 'Can you see it?' she asks.

A multi-coloured knitted leaf, the three-pronged shape of ivy, blurs in and out of focus. We talk for a while longer and she tells me she's been keeping all the doors open to let the house breathe, to let air chase out the germs whenever my brothers have visited her. As we say goodbye I wrap my arms, like wings, round the screen. She leans in, eyes glinting and I open the screen as wide as it will

11

go. Now we're hugging like un-named crows. She hangs up first and I fold my laptop screen closed.

There are many open doors and windows in her house. It used to be a Victorian school so the rooms are large and airy. A blackbird flew in through a door just before my dad got suddenly ill. It flew straight into the jaws of one of their two tabby cats. It died inside a wide-open mouth. My dad died around two months later.

All over the world there are superstitions about birds going into houses. In New Zealand, fantails come into the house to announce death, unless they fly out of the same open window they flew in. In Scotland, any bird that dies indoors predicts a death in the house. I boarded a plane three months after my dad died. Flying off chasing love. Flitting across the whole world chasing survival. If I hadn't...

Shaking off the thought, I go through to the other room. Morgan is sprawled across the sofa watching a documentary about murderers. I get a glass of wine and she shuffles herself upright so I can sit beside her.

Her voice, 'How're you, sweetheart?'

'I've got a tangle head. It'll pass.'

Her warm hand squeezes mine, an agreement to silence.

I whisper, 'Thank you, for you.'

The wine glass contains reflections of the fire. When I was fifteen, my friends and I played with a Ouija board in the room my mum was in when we spoke, the same room my dad died in five years ago. As teenagers, we'd shut ourselves in to be alone with whatever we wanted to play with.

Tonight, time doesn't feel linear. I'm in three places. One part of me is here in New Zealand with the person I love most in the whole world. Another part of me is in Scotland giving my mum a feathered crow-hug.

Another part has time-travelled away. I'm fifteen again. My dad is still alive, but he and my mum haven't yet put any silhouetted bird stickers on the tall windows. Birds often fly into them, instantly breaking their necks on a glass sky.

I am a ghost in that house. I watch a nest of teenage fingertips on an upturned glass that moves across a black Ouija board towards white letters. The glass spells out the same words over and over again in response to some question we've forgotten asking—*open close*, it spells. *Open, close.* We watch it in silence, searching for understanding, not finding it. For many years, I've wondered what that ghost meant.

But now I am back there as an adult. I am invisibly watching teenagers talking to ghosts while here, I am on the sofa beside a fire. I am controlling the movements of their glass while drinking the reflections of flames from my own. I am trying to tell them to seal up all the windows and doors so that in the future, no blackbird ever flies in and dies in that house.

I know it is too late, but I am telling them anyway. I am trying to tell them in the language of birds and ghosts:

Open, close. Open, close. Open, close.

The Places of Ghosts and Birds

People ask me, why are you in New Zealand,
so far from where you were born?
The short answer is: I came here for love.
This is truthful.
There's also a much longer answer.

It's fragmented, as stories often are
when they're difficult to tell.

This is probably where it should begin:

In Summer 2013 I left my marriage, abandoned my home,
job and possessions in Brighton,
and became voluntarily homeless.

My ex-wife Z seemed to hate it when I said, 'I don't know.'
I said it far too often. I still do, though no one mentions it any more.

When I left, I knew a lot of things
but all of them were too fast for me to see clearly.

I had too much adrenaline to stay in one place for long.

I believed I didn't deserve another home
because I'd let myself get trapped
for fifteen years inside the last one.

For months I flitted up and down the UK on trains
seeking house-sits, spare beds
any available perch.

Half-sleeping in rattling carriages, guarding my bag,
half-dreaming between locations.

My rucksack contained everything needed for comfort:

                    a cat blanket, phone charger,
        small coffee plunger, water bottle, multi-tool,
        travel sewing kit, notebook and fine-line pens,
        paintbrush, 5B pencils, laptop, calligraphy pen,
        toiletries, bright red lipstick, kindle, plasters,
                a few clothes and space for more.

I wrote thought-fragments in my notebook:

2013
Leaving Backwards

In Brighton the taxi reverses all the way
from the charity shop
which helps British hearts
bin liners and boxes are crammed
in the boot, back seat, passenger side.
The driver uncreases his frown
unfolds his arms, 'this is What'
and unsaying this question, inhales a gasp
as I hurl my possessions
into mounds on the pavement,
Road Rugby. Six number goodbye.
The letterbox spits a key into my hand
I unlock the front door and go inside
to take my wedding ring from the mantelpiece
and push it back onto my finger,
loosening it tight.

            I gathered small objects to remind me of places.
    A rose petal. A shell. A picture postcard of a convent in
                                            Lancashire.

Whenever visiting my parents in south west Scotland,
my dad and I would go for long walks.
We'd examine lichen in a glen,
or watch seabirds along a craggy shoreline.

While waves smashed against rocks
we'd listen to the deep gulps of the Irish sea.
These sounds were dark purple, sometimes brown.

I'd felt invisible for a long time,
but the year after leaving Brighton
I saw more of my parents than I had for years.
They were visible. Solid.
I'd flit away from them and back again.

Without being tied to a place, I was as free as wild birds are.

I worked wherever I could:
editing, writing, teaching creative writing.
I used money to buy time, not possessions.

I was unfixed.

For over a year, I landed in temporary places across the UK:
Cumbria. Kintyre. Argyll and Bute. Glasgow.
Cheshire. Edinburgh. Devon. Inverness. Shropshire.
Homeowners liked having someone to look after their
cats, gerbils, snake, hamsters, goldfish, plants, lawns,
while the humans were travelling.

Stone holiday cottages needed a solitary caretaker
to spread air through empty rooms, to warm
out the damp through winter months.

I kept wondering if adrenaline was addictive
and if this was dangerous or not.

I was here and not here.

Part of me was haunting the life in Brighton I'd suddenly left behind. Part of me was writing my third novel about a transient circus girl. Part of me was inventing new words.

A New Word for Loneliness

Despane– The loneliness of feeling misunderstood, unloved or unheard by someone who used to understand, love or listen.

This is how I remember it:
Before I left Brighton,
my ex-wife Z
told me she had no good memories of our relationship.

                                              Eyes stinging
           I mentioned funny conversations,
                     birthday parties in our flat.
                               Holidays:
the romance of squeezebox buskers in Paris
the red-red-red breath-sounds of their musical instruments
                         roadside cacti in Malta
                 narrow backstreets of Naples
                     art galleries in London...

Z told me
on each trip I'd said or done something that ruined it for her.
She said I couldn't remember properly,
that my memories were distorted.

      Now, I have no good memories of our relationship either
because I listed my good memories and she told me why they
                              weren't true.

          I have vague images, when searching for them:
               Of dancing at Pride, net skirt over jeans

        Z in a cowboy hat, head-thrown-back, laughing
          Erasure blaring out white-pink-green tunes,
                soaked in rain and mud.

Of my ocean circle drawing
tattooed on her shoulder.

Of Z in the shower with sunlight falling on her curly hair.
Zoom in. Water and soap suds shot through with curls and light.

Was I silent while looking at her?
She seemed to dislike not knowing what I was thinking.

This is how I remember it:
When we first met Z told me she was made of anger.
I didn't believe her, then.
Fifteen years later she cut off communication.
She'd warned me for all those years that she never stayed friends
with her exes.

Forever-silence might be her punishment to me,
I don't know
but I'm relieved there's no contact.

I've never cried about her.
That's a terrible, shameful thing,
not to cry over someone you've been with for fifteen years.

But if there are no good memories what is there to cry over?

2013
Juggler

I wear a harlequin mask
while pavemented to a spot.
Catching coins in a hat,
clothed in false jewels and
black diamonds,
I'm juggling plates exactly
as you taught me to.
I'm looking for a beam
of light to walk away on
but I see your
ghosted eyes in this crowd of smiles;
you're waiting for my hands to falter.
You're still there, now you're gone.
One plate smashes against concrete
and another, and another.

In a world without you
the sun is too bright.
My eyes can't adjust.
Thoughts are bleached white.

                              This is how I remember it:
              When the relationship was nearing the end
                    there were many late-night discussions.

I'd often shake

    and then couldn't recall exactly what had been said.
    It was probably frustrating for her.

    Z often asked me to write things down—
    so I'd know what had been agreed to
    and things she wanted me to more fully understand.

The final discussion with Z that I wrote about in my notebook:

2013
Z says our relationship is toxic.
Z has no happy memories of us.
Z doesn't want me to be happy because if I am,
I won't work at our relationship.

The things I was being told to remember were
being rejected by the places the shaking started from:
within the spine.
The cord, perhaps.
Or the marrow.

My shoulder blades picked up the tremble, deep
inside the stumps wings could have grown from.

This is what I remember
about the end of the relationship:

Z gave me an ultimatum
she must have known
was impossible—

she told me to choose between her, or writing.

A Story about Choice

Once upon a time there were two vultures who lived inside a cage in Brighton. From the outside the cage looked like an ordinary flat, in an ordinary house, on an ordinary terraced street. The vultures looked like any other loving pair who lived in Brighton.

But inside the cage one vulture wanted a lot of things it didn't have. It was getting louder and louder and bigger and bigger and the other vulture didn't want anything at all. It was getting quieter and quieter and smaller and smaller.

It was becoming cramped inside the cage.

One day, the loud vulture gripped the quiet vulture's neck with its beak.

It said, 'Choose, between me or breathing.'

The quiet vulture realised in that precise moment love had already flown out of the cage.

It also realised the cage door was open and had been open all along.

The quiet vulture chose breathing.

As the quiet vulture left the cage, it transformed into a solitary starling.

Avoiding all flocks, the starling flew away from the flat, away from the terraced street, away from Brighton. It flew as far away as it could get and then it flew away even further.

In Brighton, the loud vulture stepped out of the cage and gathered up everything it had always wanted. And then it transformed into a brightly-coloured peacock.

Neither of them had ever really been vultures.

But that is what living in a cage with someone who no longer loves you, or without all the things you want, can do.

The Cage

The human heart is a bird.
        sing by listening
   heart listen   alone.
          sing   other birds,   imitating   song.
             still   silent.   nothing to
    learn   by listening
             the closest   become
Birds   birds,
                      birds,
        contained in a
                                     song.
The human heart is a bird

      lonely

                     imitating   song.

There is much I miss about living in Brighton. I have cried over
Brighton, many times.

I miss:
knowing all the main streets, back streets, secret alleyways,
having friends I've known for a long time,
I miss being known.

    I miss:
    my family travelling to visit me in my home,
    people I didn't even like that much,
    it being easy to find jobs,
    being trusted quickly,
    going inside my friends' homes,
    friends coming into my home.

I miss:
watching the derelict West Pier disintegrating into the sea,
the swarms of starlings at dusk,
seagulls who stole sandwiches,
walking the South Downs and in the Rose Gardens and Stanmer Park.

I miss:
hearing the drummers on the pebble beach
who disappeared long before I did.
The Victorian and Regency architecture
the seafront—empty and stormy in winter.
A carousel with wild-lipped rising-falling horses and music the
colours of jelly sweets.

But I often used to walk through those Brighton streets with tears
rolling down my face.

Invisible.

I wanted someone to make eye contact with me,
to say,
'Hey, hey. Stop. Look at me. Let's talk.
What's happening, what's wrong?'

But no one did. Even if they had,
I couldn't have answered, because
everything was so wrong
no numbers added up
the alphabet went backwards
snow felt warm and sunshine was cold
and I didn't even know it at the time.

After I left Brighton, everything became strange
because I became strange.

Some friends hinted to me that I was having a breakdown.
But it wasn't about anything broken. It was about mending.

After leaving I began remembering who I was, before.
I used to like:
drawing, dancing,
listening to the same melancholic songs over and over again.
Going for solitary walks in wild weather,
watching white gulls flying beneath grey clouds in cold wide skies.
Playing the guitar and not caring if it's any good.
Watching crows flying over gold wheat fields.
Staying in the same place for long enough to learn all its textures.
Gazing up at nests in the high trees of rookeries.

Writing and writing and writing without being stopped.

Between house-sits, visits to my parents
anchored me to the ground.

My mum aired their spare room
and let me paint its terracotta walls white.
She lent me novels
played videos of murder mysteries on the telly.
She showed my hands how to knit again,
and gave me a ball of blue wool.

My dad and I visited the local wetlands.
We spied on woodpeckers
as they hopped and crawled up mossy trees.
We went down the coast to the high cliffs of the Mull of Galloway.
He was volunteering at a nature reserve
brimming with plants, insects, lichens.
A sanctuary for birds.
He wrote notes in a logbook while I walked along the cliffs.
We sat together quietly during his lunch break
then walked to craggy rocks, tiptoeing the edges of land-meets-ocean.

Seabirds dived, fished, wheeled, surfed thermals.
We watched them and talked
we watched them without speaking at all.

When I'd first moved to Brighton,
a few years before I met Z
sunlight used to sing in ice-cream colours along the seafront.
The starlings used to murmur-sing
patterns through the sky.
The drummers beat their singing drums
underneath the disintegrating pier.

I used to sing, too.
Was my singing real?
Those strange half-memories:
singing along to The Mercy Seat in a friend's living room,
Tainted Love in karaoke bars,
ancient witch-songs, sung to tides under a full moon,
my love for that moon.

Those early memories of Brighton were allowed to feel happy,
weren't they?
They were allowed to.
But for some reason, they didn't.

On one of my birthdays
I'd watched my friends drink beer,
then we went down to the seafront.
I sat on a wall and watched the starlings.
My friends played football on the lawn behind me.

I thought about the hearts of starlings, all beating as a flock.
About their hearts, singing

and wished I was up there with the starlings
instead of down here on the edge of this odd birthday.

Nothing was wrong. Nothing was right.

After Z and I broke up, I tried to go back to Brighton.

There was a kind man who wanted me to stay
but I shook whenever he touched me.

I returned and left.
Returned and left—
never stayed long enough to learn
how to stop shaking.

I said goodbye.
Stayed friends.
Stayed gone.

Whatever memories I have or don't have,
Brighton is a place I can no longer return to.

Stop Being Thistledown

though softer than air   lighter than sunshine
twisting more than other people's keys   carried pocket-deep
reminders of home, walls, doors which close and   open again
not everything can   be a trap,

stop being thistledown
because now   so afraid—
I've lost/dropped everything, gone   spinning away
on the north wind which really does blow   without snow.

stop being thistledown
after this year of nothing owned, this year of   refusals to commit,
reading no one's news. To   detach trust from
non-promise, to fly wind carried, can I   land. Is it possible?

stop being thistledown
because what do I still flee   why allow gales to decide
in this rush of missing   the travel routes
                                                                             why not choose the direction?

stop being thistledown
when at first, air seemed the only freedom   it's dizzying up here
to see light, feel temperature   there's altitude to consider

before landing to field, pavement, a beach no one goes to.

stop being thistledown
and find time's meaning again   with you, without you, with you
tear the corners off newspapers   detaching dates.

Two Words for Loneliness

Despane– The loneliness of feeling misunderstood, unloved or unheard by someone who used to understand, love or listen.

Starn– Craving something or someone to be there but knowing it's/they're not. Wanting to bite something.

Land

Over time, I reconnect online with Morgan. I first met her in 1991 when I was an art student at Dartington College of Arts in Devon. She wrote my degree course and taught there during my first year. We haven't seen each other since back then.

She lives in New Zealand.
She seems to be always awake.

I am anywhere and everywhere in the UK.
I am rarely asleep.

She is inside the words she types to me on Facebook. Then I am inside her words in private messages, soon my words breathe her words back to her in emails.She is a writer and an artist. She writes sentences that sing in colours, smells, breath, touch, sounds.

We fall in love by writing to each other

half-dreaming.

'I don't belong anywhere. I've become unfixed.'
        'Hey you. Go and get some coffee.'
'Oh, OK.' (smiling at you)
        'Talk soon, little bird.' (smiling back)

        'I'm coming over to the UK, for work.'
'Can I see you?'
        'Of course. What if we don't like each other's smells?'
'Or voices. Or something else we can't control?'
        'I've been thinking about that too.'
    'We'll keep writing, just like this.'
        'I can't bear to lose you. To lose this.'

We meet in a corporate hotel in York.

It is magical to be able to touch each other.

We eat green apples stolen from reception.

Morgan travels onwards to Chicago,
I buy a plane ticket and follow her.

We watch a tightrope walker cross a highwire.

Make up stories about an octopus and a jellyfish

and watch the night-time and day-time people

in high-rise windows.

We drink Negroni cocktails

listen to songs by Nouvelle Vague

we kiss. Again and again,

we kiss.

Morgan flies back to New Zealand.

I fly back to the UK and

land.

My dad is suddenly ill.

I fly back to the UK and

    land.

My dad is suddenly ill.

My mum meets me from the airport
drives me straight to the hospital.

I land and my dad is suddenly ill.

He is tangled in hospital sheets.
Pulled muscles.
Smaller.
Thinner.

He has been waiting for me to arrive
so he can tell both of us together.

'It might be, it might be,
it might be cancer—they're doing tests.'

We cling to hope but it is removed quickly.

My dad is dying.

While my dad is dying I need to be in one place for a while—no more than a short trainride from my parents' home near Stranraer. I persuade a landlord in Glasgow to rent me a flat for three months.

It seems impossible to call the flat a home. I don't have homes any more. But if it's out of necessity, it can be just another temporary place. As soon as I get the keys I discover far too much about the previous tenant. A never-cleaned oven. A stained mattress. A forgotten sex toy crammed between sofa cushions.

After getting a new mattress I get stuck in a loop of cleaning: of washing up liquid and bleach, cloths and scrubbing brushes, disinfectant, washing powders and scourers... Morgan is going to travel from New Zealand again to visit me here. It has to be clean. Warm. Light.

Long before she arrives, I need to show photographs of this flat to my dad. As long as he knows where I am, when he's dead his ghost will be able to come and find me. He'll need to see details. This place has to look like a proper home in the photos, so he isn't worried.

I keep cleaning, and when it still isn't clean enough I search local newspaper adverts and employ professional cleaners to finish the job. They clean it till everything is shining, but after they've gone, there are still stains in the carpet. Wearing gloves to protect my cracked hands, I keep trying, but can't work out what the stains are. Brown stains on brown carpet open up far too many possible interpretations.

My dad sends a text asking if everything is all right.

Glancing at my rucksack, I stop scrubbing and call him.

'I'm fine. Do you want me to come back tonight?'

'Tuesday,' he replies. 'You'll come back on Tuesday.'

I laugh. 'Not sooner, then?'

'Nope, Tuesday.'

On Tuesday I get the early train from Glasgow to Stranraer. My brothers are all staying there too, negotiating for moments of space and moments of togetherness. During the day, my dad's friends also come over to visit. He's become an expert at summoning people to his side. At night we gather together and do whatever he wants.

Reading a few pages from our favourite books. Playing music. Talking about memories.

I'm remembering people who were inside this house at other times too, when it was derelict. I have ghost-memories in these rooms. My dad's big-lipped mother and his blind father, visiting one summer. A broken trampoline. My little cousin as a toddler, chasing the echo-lines of shouted sounds around an empty room, long before we knew he was autistic. His sister and I chasing him, chasing sounds. My mum's parents getting ready to walk down to the shore where my dad would take their photograph on the ragged coastline. Captured forever in an oblong image, hugging each other as they gaze at a wild grey sea.

When I get some alone-time with my dad, I show him photographs of the clean flat in Glasgow. He squints at my phone, craning to see the image on the small screen. I point out the lightness of the windows and the shapes of the plants outside. The large red fireplace with its plastic coal fire. My books on the shelves. The white surfaces of the kitchenette. The leaky blue vase from a charity shop on Byers Road.

He nods when I show him my drawings of running horses, pinned on the walls. He frowns at the black curtain I've added to the white-tiled shower-room.

His eyelids droop and his hand squeezes mine.

While he's asleep. I whisper into his dreams. 'In Glasgow go to the West End—along Byers Road, near the top. Don't be too distracted by the charity shops—I'll have bought all the good treasure already. Turn left onto Huntly Gardens. Go up the hill past the church. If you're flying, have a quick look at the church roof—the architecture is gorgeously gothic. At number 31 come down to the basement and tap on the window. Day or night, don't worry about time. I'll be awake for you.'

A day later, my time with my dad comes around again. He's in a borrowed medical chair which provides support for his weakening muscles. I'm on the sofa beside him. The skin of his hand feels oddly thin. I think about how good it feels to say nothing at all. How few people can be silent together.

He says, 'I'm so glad you're settled now. A home, finally!'

Though I'm aware my sense of home is fragile, I smile as I nod. 'We're good, aren't we? Me and you?' As he looks at me, his green eyes shine with moisture.

Eye contact has always been hard for him. I meet his eyes.

Tears rise.

I am scared to blink in case he looks away.

Smiling at him, I dismiss all the arguments we've ever had. I dismiss all the clumsy or thoughtless things he could have done differently. I dismiss all the ideal-father-things I'd have liked him to have said. I dismiss the heavier things we can't easily talk about and secrets that are suddenly irrelevant.

I reply, 'We're great. We've always been great.'

He makes a contented sound, something between a hum and a sigh.

I tell him all about Morgan. He smiles as he hears we're in love and will be together, though we don't yet know how or where.

Talking gently to him, I ease his mind so he's no longer concerned about me.

Secrets of a Stitchbird (Part I)

Stitchbirds are not stitchers, or weavers, or threaders. They are called stitchbirds because their call sounds like the word, stitch. They are the only birds who mate face-to-face. Endangered, as the only member of the bird family, notiomystidae, they puzzle ornithologists.

If I was the only surviving member of my own family, I would feel endangered. I would lie low. Instead of calling or singing or crying, I could learn to become an expert stitcher, or a weaver, or a threader, by quietly watching the skilled legs of spiders. Then I could embroider the stories of my stitchbird family, to be read by future unhatched eggs. I might be tempted to sing these stories as songs while I stitched. I might be tempted to add percussion as I flurried from flower to flower, supping sugar, gathering stems for additional story-threads. I might be pulled by sound, but drawn to silence.

Back in my nest, high in an old tree, I would dream-shriek the wildest of my family's stories all through the night and invent new tales as well. In the morning, I would draw thread-words through the air between trees, pull sentences from one wire fence to another and fill empty doorways with unravelling paragraphs. These stitches would tell and untell the family stories which were unspoken or half-formed, the secrets that bound silences.

As a story-threading stitchbird, I would have a vivid life because wherever there are endangered wings, there is the possibility of dangerous flight. I would be drunk on nectar more times than I cared to remember because nectar would help me remember all the family stories I'd buried deeply in my mind. While drinking alone I would be free of all judgement. For company I would flirt with many flowers, even risqué and abundant roses, but only sip from a few. I would be intimate with bird-lovers, all feather-soft and claw-scratched, sharp-tongued and sighing. I'd be famous for demanding they look deep into my shining black eyes. 'Memorise my face,' I'd coo into their ears. 'Not the back of my anonymous neck.'

As an endangered stitchbird I would not want to be gossiped

about, stitch, stitch, stitch, while I was still alive. Trust. It's important, in one way or another, to all families. I've been a secret-keeper for as long as I can remember. There are some stories I will never tell.

Secrets of a Stitchbird (Part II)

I can't write about when   chocolate buttons   I can't tell
the story of how he woke me   when he found out   . I can't
say   that
.   he was unable to recognise   in all of their forms. I can't
he thought he was   and I don't know if   agreed with him or not. I
can't write about when he told me that   encountered.
I can't write about him not understanding   .
I can't write about how   , every morning, but he was   that
he would rather   than   . I can't express how   when
he couldn't understand   and thought it was   . I thought he was
        when   . If that had been different, I wouldn't
still feel so bad for   . He had never wanted
            . I can't write about how   he felt   and how
I can't write that this makes me   ,
discovered. It's impossible to say that   he lived and
died   ,   openly. But why then,
did
                            ? When he climbed a stone wall to look at
the full moon, he said,   and this would have made me cry
if I had known then that this conversation would always remain a secret.

39

Secrets of a Stitchbird (Part III)

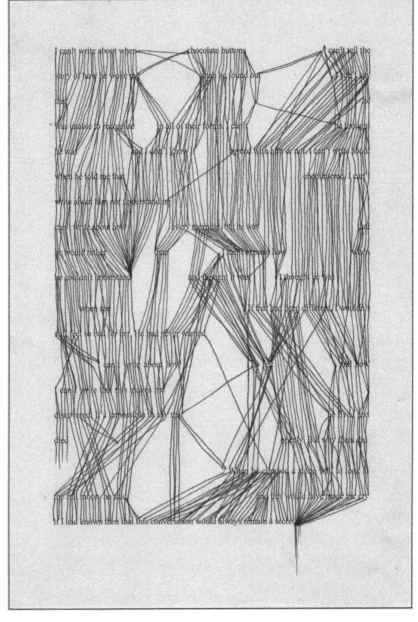

While my dad is dying,
he says, 'Love is bigger than death.'
He writes a poem telling us, his close family,
to continue to speak to him aloud when he's dead.

> Talking to someone who's dead
> is always in present tense.
> So, time changes shape.
> My memories are all in present tense
> the future is in present tense
> the present moment is vivid and intense.

While my dad is dying,
my dad's sister arrives, having driven all the way to Scotland
from the south of England.
She's crouched next to him.
He leans back in his medical chair.
She holds out her mobile phone and records his voice.

> FUTURE MEMORY:
> On the first anniversary of the day my dad died,
> my aunt re-plays the recording at her home in Kent.
> She writes to tell me what it's like to hear his voice.
> I half-read a description of emotions.
> I read them, but don't hear them.

> *Each night a pair of barn owls call, as one searches for the other*
> *in darkness.*
> *White ghosts in night.*

FUTURE MEMORY:
When my dad is dead I'll search for his ghost.
In Scotland I'll hunt through the wind-tangled branches of trees
examine the gaps between cold stars
focus my listening on the centre of wind tunnels.
In London I'll look up at the roof-edges of gothic art galleries.
At Heathrow when I wait for my plane to New Zealand,
I'll search the white lines which are drawn across the sky.

A pair of barn owls call as one searches for the other.
White feathers glide through darkest night.

My parents taught me to have no religion.
But I try to find faith, in something.
I keep repeating thoughts, words, phrases
lyrics from songs.
Repetition and echoes must be
the kinds of languages ghosts understand.

While my dad is dying,
in the garden he's tended for over forty years,
he leans on my arm while pointing at a curled shrub.
'That's witch hazel. It's my favourite tree.'
While he's busy dying,
he's telling me this for the first time.
He wants me to remember.

When waiting, tense and alert, owls rotate their heads.
They can see in all directions. Past. Present. Future.
Do they have memories or hope, or only pure instinct?
Do they dream about rain and moonlight, winter air beneath wings
or the claw-wide swoop, the kill, the blood-flavours?
Or do they dream of each other
of being together in the future.
Pairs of barn owls call to each other all through the night.

Death without religion makes past and future thoughts ache-sore.
Time remains strange.
There is no morning before
this dawn,
no predictions beyond
this night.
Time is present, static, tense,
hold tight.

While my dad is dying,
he sits beside me at the kitchen table, struggling to eat.
My mum and eldest brother are overtired.
They have gone into town
to buy him tinned custard and rice pudding.
My middle and youngest brother have gone out for a run.
My dad tells me again about the violence of his dad and asks me,
'Have I been a bad father?'

> *When I left Brighton, I forgot to take*
> *a precious box of photographs.*

While my dad is dying,
I tell him,
'You've been the best father in the world.
Ask any one of us four.'
He asks, 'Was I like my own father?'
I remember him smacking me at school
when I was a pupil in his class
but I'm pretty sure he's long forgotten this.
I reply, 'No. You didn't hurt us.'

> *A pair of barn owls cry as they swoop through darkness.*
> *White ghosts, hunting each other all night.*

Because I left the box of photographs in the Brighton flat with Z,
(who will no longer communicate with me)
I won't ever get those photographs or negatives back.
Many of them were images of my family and old friends,
places lived in, drawings made and destroyed.
There were many photographs I'd taken of my dad.

> While my dad is dying,
> he says, 'I smacked your little brothers.'
> Those smacks were my fault,
> for being upset because they'd taken
> my favourite books outside
> and covered their pages in mud.

If I hadn't cried, he wouldn't have known.
Maybe I should apologise to them sometime.
I reply, 'You did. But only once.'
'Your mum made me stop.'
'You always had choice.'

Without photographs
images of memory-scenes come loose
from their correct time and place.

MEMORY: while I am seven, eight, nine years old,
my dad shows me and my brothers
how to make valentine cards
out of white paper doilies and red card.
He tells us that this day celebrates love
and everyone in our home gets at least one card
on February the 14th.

While my dad is dying,
we talk about string-food
he is a wet-eyed little boy
until he says suddenly,
'We don't need to talk about this anymore, I'm fine now.'
I linger nearby while he finishes his meal,
chewing and swallowing,
chewing and swallowing.

MEMORY: I am six and wearing pyjamas
because it's past my bedtime.
At the kitchen table my dad gives me a dead bird.
'And here's some paper to draw on. I'll leave you to it.'
He shuts the door behind him.
I fall asleep with my face on a drawing of a swift.

While my dad is dying,
it's cold in my parents' house. and
My dad's sister is dressed
in a faux-fur edged winter shawl.

She removes her gloves and holds both my dad's hands while
they talk quietly together.
Soon she has the same child-hurt in her eyes as he does.
When the three of us are alone
I hug her and call her auntie.
This naming makes her grow up again.

> MEMORY: My dad teaches at the local primary school
> where my brothers and I are all in different classes.
> My mum's wearing a purple scarf I get teased for.
> At school I am being called gypsy-girl.
> 'Do you have to wear it?' I ask.
> My mum says, 'It doesn't matter, I like gypsies.'
> My dad tells me, 'Just ignore them. It's none of their business.'
> My dad says he'll never shave off his beard, not for anyone.
> The other kids at school call him monkey-man.
> I develop a hatred of bananas.
> The headteacher tells me,
> 'No one with a beard can ever be smart.'
> She also tells me only smart teachers
> can ever become a headteacher.
> She has long red fingernails
> and a stinging ruler.

While my dad is dying,
Morgan writes him an email telling him she loves me,
and that she'll look after me.
He writes to her in reply.
He tells me he hopes he might meet her
when she flies over in December,
but we all know he won't last long enough.

> During the days he is dying through,
> there are many repetitions of the word love.
> I say it, my mum says it,
> my dad and aunt and brothers say it.
> To each other, face to face, one at a time.
> We don't say the dead-word hope.

Doctors killed this word
and buried it far out of our reach.

MEMORY: When I'm at art college,
I sometimes visit my parents
during the breaks. I bring sketchbooks with me
 so I can show my dad drawings of birds
printed with ink and leaves and my pages and pages
of writing about being silent.
He's proud of me for going to art school.
I wish he'd been able to go to art school too,
so I make sure he learns about everything I'm learning.
I visit my parents on my dad's birthday.
He shows me his sketchbook,
filled with drawings of stones, rocks, trees.

While my dad is dying,
alone in the tiny room I'm sleeping in,
I pick mud off my splitting boots
and watch it crumble away.

MEMORY: My dad buys jewel-coloured silk shirts
from charity shops. Red. Blue. Green. Purple.
He and my mum visit me in Brighton and we joke
that he 'travels heavy' as my mum shows me her one light bag
and he brings in boxes and bags from their car.
He's brought many silk shirts with him, one for every day.
We visit charity shops together, seeking out more treasures,
filling more bags for him to take home.

While my dad is dying,
memory experienced as a present moment
is re-lived, revived, replayed, immediate.
Fragmented.
I can hear the barn owls whenever I close my eyes.
It doesn't even have to be night.

MEMORY: When I get time off from my job in Brighton,
I catch a plane from Gatwick to Scotland.
My dad and I draw pictures together.
The rules are that:
1) we're not allowed to talk at all
2) we have to take turns to
3) draw one line at a time.
Together, we draw a picture of a moon and a deer,
a landscape of trees which becomes a parrot
and a wise-looking fox under a tree.

A pair of barn owls call up the darkness.
White feathers are ghosts in a night sky made of indigo feathers.

FUTURE MEMORY:
Sometimes I make bargains—
I will never speak again until there's
a response from my dad's ghost.
I break all of my bargains all of the time.
It is winter. Many strong things become
fragile and breakable when ice spreads, banishing   warmth.

MEMORY: I'm a teenager and our home,
Dhuloch Schoolhouse,
is being haunted by something that isn't there.

While my dad is dying,
each night a pair of barn owls
cross fields, lochs and woods
to circle this house my father is dying in.
They only communicate with each other at night—
in calls and responses.

A pair of barn owls search for their own shadows in darkness.
Darker ghosts live under lake ice, which reflects cold stars.

FUTURE MEMORY:
There's ice frozen in a protective layer
all through my heart. A crack deepens.
I only know the ice is there when I feel it shift,
an earthquake of the heart.

While my dad is dying,
he is now too sick to go outside and hear the owls,
so listens from his chair.
The barn owls don't know which direction to fly in,
unless there's a response to their call.

FUTURE MEMORY:
I hold ice-cubes in my palm
while wondering if ghosts speak in a language
of echoes, rhythms, repetitions?
We don't need as many humans around us as we think.
Just one or two, perhaps a few occasionally. The ones who care.
There are so many who don't.
Look away.
Gone.

A ghost calls, searching for another ghost in darkness.
Soft call, tu...wit. Softer response, tu...whoo.

FUTURE MEMORY:
At this kitchen table if I draw all the birds
my dad ever saw when he was alive,
will the ghosts of those birds bring him to me?

While my dad is dying,
anyone who can still eat
gathers at the kitchen table for meals,
often cooked by his friends.
In this raw time together,
I can only speak of now,
trying to repeat the best alive-words.
The bright-or-light coloured words with the gentlest sounds.

48

These familiar words are needed:
big moon. Kindness. Stars. Love.
Sunshine. Gratitude. Owls. Fresh air.

One day, the past and the future might
return to their correct places.
The whole world
is full of love and death.
These two enormous forces are of equal size.

While my dad is dying,
barn owls circle
and call
and circle.

Beneath the southern cross,
my wife calls to me from the future.
Through dark clouds I call back.

Soft call, ho...pe. Softer response, ho...pe.

Three Words for Loneliness

Despane– The loneliness of feeling misunderstood, unloved or unheard by someone who used to understand, love or listen.

Starn– Craving something or someone to be there but knowing it's/they're not. Wanting to bite something.

Youache– Where a specific person is missed and only their physical presence will cure the ache of missing them.

My father dies at the age of sixty-seven on the 9ᵗʰ of December
2014, surrounded by my three brothers, me, and my mum.

While holding his hand
I watch death happen to him.
All of us speak words to him
and all of us are silent.

> I love my three brothers and mum so much in this moment
> but I can barely look at them.
> I'm staring at them.
> I can barely look at them.
> My mouth says things that are important.
> My mouth says nothing.

I will never speak of watching death.
(I'm still holding his hand. I can't let go.)

> *You don't see us at the window bright-eyed*
> *looking in at you all*
> *three sons, a daughter, a wife*
> *the dying watcher in his chair.*
> *We perch on the branches of trees he planted*
> *and sing our favourite song.*
> *The one that goes: you-never-heard-us-singing.*

My dad is a teacher, an artist, photographer, musician,
a campaigner for nuclear disarmament, a gardener, a birdwatcher
just before he died, he volunteered at a bird-sanctuary.

> *We fly away and back twice, thrice,*
> *to catch him out in our counting joke.*
> *How high, how low. How long?*

Do the birds notice he is no longer here?
Perhaps he is with the birds.

Too soon too soon, not yet not yet.

Perhaps that is exactly where he is.
Haunting their wings
practicing flitting from one to the other,
possessing each one. What do the birds think?

Who allows a human ghost inside their heartcage
to beat the body into flight?
Do not fill us with your ghosts. We are carrying our own.

Travel-by-bird would be the kind of thing he'd try.
I imagine him getting used to the flutters of small wings,
crashing, flying, falling.

Come outside and walk along muddy roads,
sodden fields, slippery rocks along the coastline.
Leave scratches instead of footprints.

Outside, I tell the gales, 'He isn't really dead,
he's just somewhere else.'
I tell the gales, 'He'll come back.
Just a little more time and he'll come back.'

Gales steal the thing you most want,
and travel with it.

The Human Heart is a Bird

Your heart is a bird who powers your human body. This bird flaps its wings constantly, moving blood, oxygen, nutrients to every cell, nerve, and vital organ.

The bird is agitated while awake. When it sleeps, it dreams deeply. It dreams you are a scarlet room. It dreams of your pulsing walls and velvet chambers. Most of all, it dreams of flying outside of you, of escaping through your opening-closing trap doors.

The bird lives in your chest between your lungs, slightly to the left. Inside your rib cage. It feels, and is, trapped. The bird is the size of your clenched fist.

While the bird flaps its wings it sends electrical signals through your blood. These signals move oxygen around your body and to and from, your lungs.

Oxygenated and de-oxygenated blood is exchanged like waves in your capillaries because the trapped bird is trying so hard to break out of you.

Your body dies.

You become completely still.

The bird is suddenly calm and becomes completely still too. It eyes your capillaries, veins, arteries.

Your mouth is slightly open. The bird can fly out of your dead body whenever it wants to. But without its wing-flapping panics, it feels heavy as a rock.

It eyes your lungs, trachea, esophagus. Just to see if it can make you move even when its wings aren't flapping, the bird blows air through all your tubes.

It waits. Your body doesn't move. The bird forgets to breathe. Your body still doesn't move. The bird remembers to breathe. The bird sings.

It sings of all the sunsets you never saw and it sings of the clouds you never plunged through. It sings of the loves you sent flitting away, and the one you kept. It sings of your wing-envy. It sings of a humming moon you once heard but couldn't believe in. It sings of the cracking sound of all the eggs you ate but never hatched. It sings of all the twigs you broke under your heavy boots but never built nests with. It sings of the oceans you never migrated across. It sings of a great wave that grabbed a small stone, just for the sake of drowning it.

The bird sings about itself, trapped deeply inside the cage of your chest.

It sings of a body that trapped a bird inside itself because it needed a heart that could sing.

And while the bird quietly sings, its song moves like breath through all the tubes of your body. You become an instrument. It plays all the songs you would have loved, but never heard. These are melancholic sounds, sometimes cello notes bowed in a minor key, sometimes distant flutes.

The notes of this song are just above silence, or just below it.

These are the sounds of your ghost.

Travelling Light

Morgan comes over from New Zealand to stay with me for six weeks. The basement flat in Glasgow becomes our first home together. She makes a Christmas tree out of wire coathangers, educates me about proper custard, kisses me a lot and holds me in her strong arms.

She travels down to Stranraer with me to meet my whole family for the first time as we gather for my dad's funeral. My brothers and mum have arranged everything.

There are flowers all over my mum and dad's house. Time and days blur together. I don't know who sent all these flowers and more arrive yesterday and tomorrow and now the doorbell rings again. Lilies. White roses. Pale carnations. While the rest of my family collate and read the tiny cards that come with the flowers, I'm either with Morgan or on my own.

'I'm so glad she's got you,' my mum says to Morgan, again and again. 'So glad.'

When alone I walk along muddy roads, through sodden fields, along the slippery rocks of the coastline through storms and gales. I tell the storms everything I can't say out loud. I tell the gales I'm no use to anyone. The storms take away the sound of my voice and smudge it grey, black, deepest blue. I repeat over and over again, 'He's not really dead, he's just somewhere else'. Rain runs through my hair and the wind blows my face till it burns. The whole sky is filled with the sounds of whirring. Dreams are as real as these storms. These storms are dreamlike.

At the funeral, my three brothers stand next to each other and share a reading of a poem. They are beautiful seen together like this. Three very different faces, so strong and so vulnerable. I can still see the boy each of them was.

They are inches away from his wicker coffin which our mum has threaded with leaves and flowers.

When it's my turn, I stand where they stood.

I read this to my dead father:

Travelling Light

You told me in so many ways that love is stronger than death.
What I didn't realise before, was that death had such strength in its
darkness.

It had weighty shadows and each of them had momentum. They
were the waves of an unfamiliar ocean. I knew there were cliff edges.
I saw you look over them.

Unfamiliar oceans surely couldn't be conquered by anyone who'd
never travelled them before.

So where was the ship, the navigator, the captain, the crew, what
dangers could be predicted? Where were the charts, the map, the
compass?

I wanted to give you all of these things to take with you, but my
hands were empty.

There was weight and strength and momentum in death. It seemed
tidal.

You never said you were afraid, but I thought part of you must
be, because this was an unknowable journey.

While you were dying, you said you were having the time of your
life.

I realised it didn't matter what I thought at all. You were embracing
death. You were making your own preparations for this unknown
journey.

Your eyes were beautiful and strange since you became ill.

I watched your eyes all the time. Your eyes were consuming love.
It seemed to me as if you were filling yourself from a different ocean.
You didn't want the dark ocean I saw in death, but were inventing
your own. Your ocean was a place of unbearable brightness and
love—a sea made from weightless reflections and waters which tasted
of sweetness as much as they tasted of salt.

You watched wild birds and their flitting movements filled your
eyes. You looked at the people surrounding you and their love for
you filled your eyes. Your hands bruised themselves drumming, as
music filled your eyes as much as it filled your ears.

All of this love was weightless and so bright.

And when you looked at me across the kitchen table, your eyes held mine. I rolled sorrow-filled tears and you streamed joy-filled tears in response. If there was no end to sorrow, there was no end to your joy. Both of us were carrying oceans which needed to be travelled.

You were facing an unfamiliar ocean by gathering an ocean of your own.

You always packed a ridiculous amount—far too many things—whenever you were going away. Of course, for this journey, you'd pack a whole ocean. But to ride the waves of your own bright ocean, you need to be travelling light.

I've been collecting some of your light things, in case you forgot to take them all. Here's a few, just for now:

the illumination within clouds in your photographs of sunsets

the intake of breath from your primary school students as you scared them with ghost stories

the torch beam you shone across the road when we went to get milk from the farm in the night

the autumn leaves blown from every tree you ever planted

the sound of each page turning in all the books you read

the fine lines in pale pastel which completed your drawings

the broken eggshell that each seabird you counted at the Mull of Galloway hatched from

the surface reflections of all the lakes you ever stood quietly beside.

And if I could give you any gift, it would be an invisible compass that shows the direction of the heartbeat of anyone who loves you.

Love doesn't weigh a thing. Keep travelling light.

I worry about holding onto Morgan too tightly but she is the one who grabs and holds me when I try to run away from my dad's open grave.

After the funeral, time slows again. I feel guilty because I haven't done anything at all about the paperwork or arranging the funeral. My brothers and mum reassure me that I've done things they couldn't do. I can't remember what those things are, even when they remind me.

It isn't going to be easy for Morgan when she gets home to New Zealand. Back in Glasgow we clutch each other's hands as we walk through the Botanic Gardens. Extending our walk, we lean on a bridge looking down into the River Clyde.

'Look,' she says. 'The colours!'

The river is dark tonight, muscular and alive. 'Come on, artist.' I say, nudging her elbow with mine. 'Tell me.'

Frowning, she stares into the water. 'Indigo under Antwerp Blue. Burnt Umber. A tiny brushstroke of Hookers Green. Oh. And Paynes Grey.'

I love watching her finding paintings in the landscape around her. And now she's told me the colours, I can see her painting of the river overlaying the real river.

I ask her, 'If you had a fishing rod, where would you be standing, to catch a fish?'

She points to a spot further up the bank, beneath some trees. 'Somewhere around there where the water flows deep, but slow.'

And now I can imagine her standing there, dressed in blue, fishing in her own painting of this river.

As we walk along a row of brightly lit shops she glances at me with a small smile. 'I wish we were kissing, right now.'

I pull her into a doorway and kiss her.

We kiss in many doorways.

I ask her about the things she loves most: writing and fishing, reading and painting. She tells me about her own father's death while she makes a watercolour painting of the wrought iron fence and plants outside our window.

She makes me laugh and doesn't try to stop me when I cry.

Before Morgan departs I book a flight for a long visit to New Zealand in March. After she's gone we keep writing to each other from Scotland and New Zealand.

I walk the streets of Glasgow late at night and sing along with buskers if they'll let me. I smile at passing strangers who look sad. I pick up small things people have dropped and try to find their owners. A key. An empty wallet. A polkadot scarf. I sit in corners of cafes and watch groups of other people talking. Travelling by train, I visit my mum, get some of my dad's artworks framed, and come and go from the flat in Glasgow.

I take one of my dad's pastel drawings to his sister. She's away from her home in Kent, so I get on a train to Cornwall to find her and my cousins. They're on holiday in a gleaming white hotel with landscaped lawns. I've never stayed anywhere as grand as this before. We drink too much white wine. She says things she forgets she's said and I forget saying all kinds of something or nothing. No matter. No regrets.

In Wellington, Morgan is now living in a rented flat, gradually gathering things that make it feel like a home. She's building a nest out of cotton bedlinen, kitchen knives, patterned mugs. Thick towels, guitars, watercolour paints.

On Byers Road I find an empty blue suitcase leaning next to a bin. I take it back to the flat. Splayed open on the floor, it looks like the cover of a vast book with no pages. The suitcase becomes an idea collector—it is home, it is travel, it is distance, it is a collector of future-possibilities. It is a ghost-carrier. It is a small library of invisible books. It is being met from a long flight by Morgan who will miraculously bring a trolley to wheel it home. She will somehow always have known that I will arrive with a broken blue suitcase. The empty suitcase is never really empty. It keeps me company while I'm either talking to my dad or talking into the air.

My dad's ghost doesn't visit me in Glasgow. I keep talking to him but he doesn't reply. While waiting for his voice I light candles, whisper, sing, sleep or stay awake for too long, wear myself out walking too far or too fast, forget to eat, listen so hard I can't hear anything at all, play loud music to calm down the listening, call his name and cry.

I remember being a teenager. Lighting candles. Summoning ghosts again, and again.

He doesn't appear.

When the lease ends I have the option to renew it, but don't.

There's no reason to tie myself to a home my ghost dad doesn't visit.

I am unfixed again.

But there is a change—I am no longer flitting away. I am flitting towards. Morgan becomes the only fixed point on an expanding map.

If my dad's ghost can't find me in Glasgow, what if he also can't find me in New Zealand? There is no sign, message, symbol. No whisper, no co-incidence, no moment of revelation. But perhaps it's too soon. There's a delay, while he gets used to being dead. While he learns how to be a ghost. So, I'll keep looking for him wherever I am in the world.

When he's ready, when he's adjusted and gained skills in travelling, he'll come.

But in their home near Stranraer, my mum feels him holding her hand. Again and again she feels him holding her hand, or holding her. Or maybe she only tells me about this once and all the other times are an echo in my head.

She needs this so badly.

It's wives who have the strength to pull their spouses back to them after death. Daughters might try, but fail. Daughters are far too flighty to chase around the world for, especially when they're glowing with new love.

I'm hoping that once a certain amount of time has passed, geography is of no significance to ghosts. After all, they must need time to learn how to fly, or figure out how to possess the living.

Perhaps he's possessing that bird who's sitting on my mum's tiled roof right now.

When I close my eyes I can half-dream it.

A bedraggled starling, exactly the size of my clenched hand.

Summoning Ghosts

In this memory, I'm sixteen. I'm in a vodka-swirl, I'm party-avoidant, voice-drained, ears-overflowing, eyes locked onto speckled-glass. Outside this dark bedroom, the party's warming. My friends are having a great time.

Mmcha. Mmcha. Mmcha. Smash. Laughter. Bang. Mmcha. Mmcha. Mmcha.

They won't notice that tonight I don't believe in friends. Tonight, I'm more interested in believing in ghosts. The only light comes from a candle flame. I whisper into the dressing table mirror, 'So, where are you, then?'

Mmcha. Mmcha. Mmcha. Bang. Laugh-shriek. Bump. Mmcha. Mmcha. Mmcha.

My friends and I don't drink to have fun. We drink to get drunk. We drink and get damaged and try not to feel the damage. They're partying throughout the house. I'm alone in this bedroom with the light off and a chair wedging the door shut. Boys and dark rooms— bad combination. Y tried to grab me earlier, but I fought him off and got away.

When I leave this room I'll drink enough vodka to pass out till the party is over. This room won't be private for much longer— someone will want to have sex in here.

Mmcha. Mmcha. Mmcha. Thump. Shriek. Thud. Mmcha. Mmcha. Mmcha.

I focus on the candle flame. Who said I should try this spell? Now I've remembered I want to try it, vodka has increased the urgency. Was it intense-eyed Y or lace-gloved W? No, they'll be in the kitchen obsessing about what's more valuable—virginity or sexual expertise. Was it pretty V or passionate U or parrot-earringed T? No, they'll be in the front room dancing with each other. Was it camp S or deep R? Not Q. He only thinks about W. It might have been R—he's deep because he's adopted. He only thinks about W too. No. It wasn't R's voice that said—

If you light a candle and look at yourself in a mirror for long enough without blinking, you'll see a ghost.

It could have been one of the occult books I borrowed from the library. Now I think about it more, it was definitely a book. A silent ink-voice. The quietness of turned pages. I also remember reading:

If you ever see a doppelgänger—a ghost who is a double of yourself—you'll die.

Doppelgängers are only dangerous under certain circumstances. If they get drunk at one party and you get drunk at another party, it's probably fine.

It's the act of *seeing* which is dangerous.

I'm going to stare into this mirror without blinking till I see a ghost. The candle flickers, casting shadows on my eyelids.

Mmcha. Mmcha. Mmcha. Voice-mix. Laughter-shriek. Crunch-yell. Mmcha. Mmcha. Mmcha. Voice-mix. Voice-mix. Voice-mix. Why do people have to speak? *Mmcha. Mmcha. Mmcha.*

If I see a ghost maybe my hair will turn white. When people see the effects of great shock, they probably won't expect me to talk about it. Then, I'll be able to get away with being completely silent for the rest of my life. If I don't talk I won't care too much about anything, because I'll be free. I'll be calm all the time. I tried being silent once, for a whole day and night. It felt amazing. I was happy and everything was so funny. It was like living in a remarkable parallel world with no rules.

Someone bumps along the hallway outside. Y's voice. 'Anyone seen Jess?'

Shit. I didn't think they'd notice.

A door slams. Water, running. An antiseptic smell. The candle flickers. Only my mascara-soaked eyelashes are dark. My skin is bandage-coloured in candlelight. I pinch out three of my eyelashes and make three wishes. 'Help me, help me not. Help me.' I blow the eyelashes away, not quite knowing what I'm wishing for. I stare without blinking. Saltwater leaks from my eyes. My face slips, becoming two layers.

An old ghost-face looks out at me through my young face.

It's my own face, looking at me from the future.

I say, 'How old will I be when I'm finally allowed to stop talking?'

My double face is thin fabric—two faces warping, wefting.

My voice sounds shrill. 'How old?'

The old face is calm, as if it hasn't spoken for a long time.
As if there's no need to.
An elbow thuds against the door. A voice. 'Has anyone seen Jess?'
I blow out the candle and my ghost-face disappears into darkness.
No. No one's seen me.

Four Words for Loneliness

Despane– The loneliness of feeling misunderstood, unloved or unheard by someone who used to understand, love or listen.

Starn– Craving something or someone to be there but knowing it's/they're not. Wanting to bite something.

Youache– Where a specific person is missed and only their physical presence will cure the ache of missing them.

Ignornly– The kind of loneliness that other people notice, but don't mention to the person they think is lonely. Their expression shows sympathy, but also a little wariness, as if loneliness could be contagious.

Migrations

People I meet in New Zealand often ask, politely, how I ended up on this side of the world. As opposed to the other side. People in the UK often ask why I'm living on the other side of the world. New Zealand is not my birth-side. Not the everyone-I-know-lives-somewhere-I-can-easily-find-them-side. New Zealand is the believe-in-love-again-and-learn-to-think-of-the-future-and-not-death-side.

The right side, to those who are drawing side-lines, is whichever side we are standing on while we are talking. We all say it, but really, any conversation about *sides* is ridiculous. Flat-earth ridiculous. The world is a globe. A globe doesn't have *sides*, it has curves.

On my first visit to Morgan, I realise my dad would have loved New Zealand. While awake with jet lag listening to the strange calls of dawn birds, I try talking to him but there's no reply.

The first evening after I've arrived, Morgan says, 'Come on, let's go outside. I want to show you something.' She leads me down to the shore and we walk along the pavement around the coast road. The grey rocks look like the west coast of Scotland, where I grew up. I ask her about them.

She replies, 'They're greywhacke.'

'But how can the exact same type of rocks be both here and there, when the distance is so great—'

Morgan stops walking and glances at me. She's waiting for me to notice something.

I pause, inhaling. A strange scent mixed with the smell of the ocean.

She nods. 'Can you smell it?'

'It's smoky. Like nothing I've smelled before. Like earth, burning. Brown, grey, burgundy. Like grass as well. But dark, tall grass.'

Her eyes light up. She gestures at a giant flax plant with grey-green leaves and dragony flowers. All along the roadside they're punctuating the coastline between rocks. 'I wanted you to smell New Zealand. Have you caught the scent?' She beams at me and I can see how much she loves this coastline. This city. This country.

'It's beautiful,' I reply, taking her hand. 'You've brought me to a beautiful place.'

Her face glows as she grabs me and pulls me close.

'Come on, you.' I say, when we disentangle ourselves. 'Let's get some chips and eat them on the beach.'

'Fuck, I love you,' she says.

'For liking chips?' I laugh.

'Yup. For liking chips.'

On my second visit I have a working visa instead of a tourist one and haven't booked a return flight. I have a new white suitcase on wheels. Neither Morgan nor I can drive, so we walk or get buses all around Wellington. She says I'm bedraggled because I've flown such a long way. When I'm with her I feel loved. I feel love. But when I'm alone, sometimes I feel like a lost starling come loose from a flock, but landing in a beautiful place. I'm not sure how to start conversations with new people so I usually don't. Maybe I'll learn, over time. After all, everyone seems friendly here. While Morgan's working I wander the streets of Newtown, Lyall Bay, Island Bay, Kilbirnie, seeking out the twisted branches and dark leaves of Pōhutukawa. These are the trees of fairy tales.

Morgan buys a small half-a-house in Berhampore, a quiet suburb in Wellington. We move in and paint the bedroom walls white. Out in the back garden I tell my dad he'd be enchanted by the petrol-coloured feathers of tūī and their double-voiced vocabularies. I tell him to look through my eyes and watch the tiny fantails flitting everywhere, the pīwakawaka. They're made of magic and they're messengers between the living and the dead. I ask them to take him my love and if they can, bring him to visit me. I ask them if he's hitched a ride in their bodies, as they flash and dance their fans around the delicate leaves of our kōwhai tree.

They answer me with shrill cheeps and a flipping-flupping tail dance, but I can't translate their language of joy.

He never answers at all.

While Morgan and I fill the garden with tomato plants and pin new drawings and watercolour paintings on the white walls, I still keep telling him about all the things he'd love if he was here for a visit.

I watch for his footprints in wet sand, across dry rocks, on

66

pavements. New Zealand is twelve hours ahead of the UK. People in the UK think New Zealanders live in the future. I'm becoming convinced that ghosts have no interest in the future. New Zealand doesn't seem as haunted as the UK is.

But still I try to talk to him. Most of all, I tell him about Morgan. He'd have loved Morgan. He'd love her for being exactly the person she is, he'd love her for loving me, he'd love her because I love her and he'd love her for being my home.

He never speaks back.

All around me birds behave in flighty birdlike ways. I'm certain I would recognise him if he possessed one of them.

I try to find him while I'm asleep.

I dream of a wooden ladder.

I dream of climbing this ladder.

Climbing this ladder to the top of a tall and narrow tree, I look into a nest.

Inside the nest is a miniature storm. A weather-bomb. Black clouds. Lightning. Flash floods.

In the heart of the storm, opening-closing beaks greet me with small screams.

Three naked blackbird chicks, made of skin and hunger.

I examine their blind eyes and the creases of bald heads, seeking familiarity.

Which one is my dad's ghost possessing?

Not that one.

Not this one.

Not the other one.

One day, I can't see anything clearly because there's a sad-filter over my eyes. I walk down to Island Bay. Sitting on a concrete block I stare out to sea. This beach is on the other side of the world to my dad's grave. I imagine throwing flowers for him into this ocean. Carving his name into this sand and watching the waves smooth it away. Writing him a message in a bottle and sending it out to sea.

Today I am so lost, without him.

A brown dog approaches me, followed by a silver-haired man in a bluish jacket. The dog sniffs my hand and wanders off. The man says, 'Are you all right?'

'I'm fine.' I reply, wondering what he wants.

But suddenly I realise I might not look fine. My eyes are swollen from crying and a bootlace has come undone and my shirt is unevenly buttoned. There are other people scattered in small groups all along this beach. Jandalwearers. Barefooters. It's summer and I'm wearing boots as I always do, but that's probably inappropriate. I must look like an unstable loner. Heavy-booted enough to drown. Staring out to sea at the most violent waves.

'You're English,' he says.

I shrug. 'Sort of. Maybe more Scottish. A bit Welsh but not really.'

'English voice. Been here long?'

'Not long.' I reply.

His pale shorts are line-creased down the front because someone else has ironed them for him. He's wearing white schoolboy socks and sandals. He might be a born-again Christian who's wanting my tormented soul for Jesus. Do they have born-again Christians here and do they hate lesbians too, like in the UK? There's so much I still don't know.

I say, 'Thanks for your worry, but I'm not going to drown myself or anything.'

'Why d'you come here?'

'For love.'

'Ah.' He nods. Migration-for-love is a common thing, to kiwis. He says quietly, 'He didn't travel to you.'

I don't know how homophobic he might be. Instead of replying in defence of a fictitious male lover, or telling him I had no home for my lover to travel to, I stare out to sea again. Morgan says this all the time—*strangers might ask me questions, but I don't owe them the truth.*

His dog's disappeared. I wonder when he'll notice.

'You live here?' I ask, 'With your family?'

He nods.

'Are you happy?'

'Of course.'

'I'm glad. This bay is beautiful.' I glance offshore at the jagged rocks of the island.

He shifts from one foot to the other, looking at his own footprints. 'Takes at least three years, I'm told. Though everyone *seems* friendly enough.'

'What takes three years?'

'To make friends here.'

'Oh. That's quite a while, then.' I'm already doubling the number of years to six in my mind, because I'm imagining other immigrants with kids at school, sociable jobs, with religious gatherings, active nightlives. Invitations and parties and outings in groups... all the things I don't really want. Maybe it'll be more like nine years for me. Or even twelve. I can't imagine the world in twelve years. This beach, the dunes and the nearest row of houses, might be drowned underwater.

'You'll be right,' he says. 'In about three years.' He nods at me. He's kind. Just someone who lives here checking on me for looking a bit vulnerable. No agenda.

I smile at him and mean it. 'Where's your dog?'

He glances along the beach. 'Ah. In the dunes again. Best get her.'

'Thanks for talking to me. I'm a bit homesick today is all. It'll pass.'

'No worries.'

He strides off, shrilling a whistle that's palest blue. The brown dog comes bounding down the sand and leaps up at him. He loops a leash around her neck and walks away along the beach.

This country looks familiar in so many places, but then suddenly I notice a detail that seems off-kilter. Like oak trees. They don't grow tall or wide here. Their leaves look dry. Some of them have small plastic triangles strapped to a branch, traps for a particular kind of moth. There are also box-traps containing poison that kills rats and stoats, because they eat native birds. I never look inside traps.

The flax plants are unfamiliar in ways I can understand. They have muscular leaves, smoke-scented flowers. Birds flock to them, drinking their dark nectar. They fit this climate. They fit their spaces under this open sky full of overwhelming sunlight. They belong here.

When I get home, I set the kettle to boil. Morgan's outside on the deck taking a break from reading a PhD thesis. It starts spitting with rain so she comes into the house. While I spoon coffee into the plunger, I tell her about the man on the beach, about him checking on me.

She frowns and says, 'You're unhappy here.'

'No, I'm a bit sad today is all. I was telling you about him because—'

'It's my fault you're here.'

'I'd feel like this whether we were somewhere-or-other in the UK or here or any other place.' I get two mugs out of the drawer.

She leans against the kitchen counter. 'I feel bad.'

'You've got nothing to feel bad about. We decided I'd come to you because it made sense. You have a job. Friends and colleagues. I didn't have anything apart from you and writing. So I could be anywhere as long as you were there. And I can write here. You want me to write.' I rub her back.

She straightens up. 'You're so sad, though.'

I push the plunger through the grains. 'I get sad. I got sad far more often when I was still in the UK.'

She looks down at her bare feet. 'Yes.'

'So, it's not your fault, is it.'

She squeezes my hand.

I kiss her. 'Come on. Let's have this coffee. Where do you want to sit?'

She glances at the window. 'It's stopped raining.'

As I pour the coffee and get the milk out of the fridge I say, 'So anyway, this man. He checked on me. He didn't have to. So many times when I lived in Brighton I'd be alone on the seafront. I'd be feeling sad among all these groups of people sitting around, talking easily and seeming to really care for each other. I believed I was invisible. That if I walked into the sea and didn't walk back out again, no one would have seen me leave.'

She picks up her mug and takes it outside to the garden. 'There are good people here. They help each other out.'

I follow her down the steps. 'And that's a beautiful thing. That's why I was telling you about the man. I wanted to say that kiwis are kind.'

She sits on the bench under the grapevine and smiles up at me. 'I remember that list of loneliness you wrote. You posted it online and everyone on your Facebook page was saying how beautiful it was and talking about which type of loneliness they had. I wanted to yell at them, do something, people! Can't you see what she's saying? Can't you see her?'

I nudge her knee with mine. 'But now *you* see me.'

Warm into Cold

I sink myself in dreams. Neither-here-nor-there places.

I've been trying to dream in different ways and each of these methods takes me to a strange place where I might find my dad. I go lower and lower into the thickest dreams, but wake before I get deep enough to find out what's there. These deeply submerged places might be the only locations I can find him.

They might be dangerous. I might forget how to be awake.

It's only while I'm half-dreaming that my dad appears as a ghost or as a bird, or some kind of hybrid feathered-man. Sometimes I appear in my own dreams as a ghost or a bird, flitting to a strange location, flitting away again, hunting something I can never find, flitting back.

Now I'm living with Morgan, I am pulled from these dreams and unfixed places back into the real world.

Love does that. It glows, pulls and holds.

While he was alive, my dad told me a lot of stories about his life and often told me about his dreams. I thought he was brave when he spoke about painful things. Now, remembering his pain hurts. I can't speak about the private things which made him vulnerable, but I know what they were. I thought I was being brave in return, to tell him my own personal stories, but now wish I hadn't in case my pain hurt him too.

I wish all the painful stories I've ever told my dad could be unspoken, so if I caused him pain, it is undone. Sometimes pain swirls all around me and I wake soaked in sweat, screaming at the force of nightmares. In dreams, the past and present never stay in their correct locations. Sometimes I shake. Morgan holds me until I'm still again.

Through everything that's happened, she's kept me alive. I think she knows this.

My dad used to photograph birds and landscapes all along the west coast of Scotland. I have his digital camera now. Before he died, he told my mum he wanted me to have it.

I place my eye where his eye was. To see what his living eye saw. I haven't been able to change the filter settings.

He's left me a camera that gives every photograph the tinge of a yellow-pink sunset.

As I photograph the south coast of New Zealand's North Island the colours of my images come out all wrong. In the northern hemisphere, the skies are overlaid with whiteness. I miss the bright northern sky, but here, my dad's camera settings make sense.

He was bringing warmth into coldness.

I am far less haunted than I was while my dad was still alive. I'm more fixed. I don't flit. Or get myself too lost.

Though I love the home Morgan and I are making together, it isn't the building, or the place that I come back to. No matter how far I wander, she is my one fixed point, my home.

I read some more of the fragments in my notebook. I'd forgotten about the storm:

2014
The day my father, the birdwatcher, dies

I walk away from the smell
of garlic frying—hunting weather,
I stamp into this storm,
calling the crows to fly with me
into rain, gusts, gale, eye.

My arms without wings are unboiled bones—
held out to give the crows something pale
something unbroken
to fly beneath
as I call up the ravens, swifts, gannets, kites,

house martins, jackdaws, one magpie,
sparrows, starlings and herring gulls—
all the spring birds are here too
though it's deep winter.

I've got these birds up and spinning
while I call for an eagle
to fly beside me.
Wail. Whirl. Cry.

If it rains for ten years
all of the birds will refuse to fly in gales,
instead choosing
to sit in clumps and mimic rocks.
No one will go to church any more
roofs leak
no one will put umbrellas up indoors; it's bad luck
everyone's watch will be damp—
condensation flowers
stopping the ticks.

A storm called a weather-bomb
explodes
the day I watch cancer eat my father;
a vortex spreading blackness, feathering him
from within.

My dad is with me, just once, in a dream.

In this dream he's in Brighton, sitting beside me on a bench in a rose garden we often visited when he came to stay.

I lean my head on his shoulder for a while.

He glows. His glow makes me glow.

We talk quietly for a while, saying nothing of significance. Feeling it, instead.

Seagulls wail, making us look upwards. All of our words fall away as he rises to his feet, climbs onto the bench and places his camera to his eye. He silently photographs seabirds flying towards a spreading sunset.

Yellow and pink sunlight falls on his upturned face.

In this dream I've been waiting so long for, he is no more dead or alive than I am. He is just in a place I can't go back to.

Weather Bomb

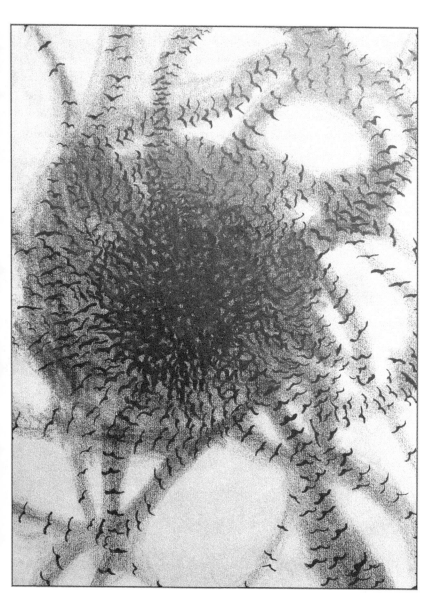

Vortex I

Cold into Warm

Morgan and I get married for the first time in New Zealand. A waiata is sung by one of Morgan's esteemed Māori colleagues at our wedding ceremony. It brings tears to all of our eyes. We laugh at the incongruous photograph of the queen which hangs on the wall in the registry office. Morgan's friends and work colleagues are at the wedding party. My friends P and O who are from the UK but live in Auckland and a friend-of-a-UK-friend I've met recently have come along. Sixty people in a room are a tangle of clashing colours, smells, lines, light reflections, textures, increasing noise and simultaneous-speaking sounds.

I focus on Morgan.

She looks beautiful in her blue clothes, her gloves and boots. A bit like a pirate. A bit like a scamp.

I'm wearing a bright red dress. We are the colours of jewels.

And there is music.

We dance to a song about belonging to each other.

None of our relatives are here.

Morgan and I

                                 are the colours of jewels.

                        belonging to each other.
                        here.

Morgan and I travel back to the UK and get married for the second time at my mum's house in Scotland. A celebrant binds our hands together with a blue and red plaited cord, handfasting us in an ancient Celtic ritual. Both our families and many old friends are here and the party lasts into the early hours. The ones who are missing—the two dead fathers, long-gone grandparents, missing aunts and uncles—are remembered but not discussed. At the end of the night, my sister-in-law wants to dance, so I turn up the music and all three of us dance until we're too tired to move our legs any more.

Morgan and I   get married   time a
                    ritual   and
            hours. The ones
                                            remembered   the end of the night
                    to dance
                                    the music and   dance

Morgan and I

                                    music and   dance

Five Words for Loneliness

Despane– The loneliness of feeling misunderstood, unloved or unheard by someone who used to understand, love or listen.

Starn– Craving something or someone to be there but knowing it's/ they're not. Wanting to bite something.

Youache– Where a specific person is missed and only their physical presence will cure the ache of missing them.

Ignornly– The kind of loneliness that other people notice, but don't mention to the person they think is lonely. Their expression shows sympathy, but also a little wariness, as if loneliness could be contagious.

Solilone– A type of melancholia experienced while gazing at a wide-skied landscape. A longing for strangeness, for the unreal or the surreal to appear.

Unsolved Memories

Poltergeists are often associated with children or teenagers. It's possible they're manifestations of an agitated and developing soul. A poltergeist might also be thought of as an imprint or an image that has been left behind. An image of an unsolved memory, replaying. This image could be reanimated by the kinds of energetic disturbances children and teenagers cause. The five memories described below can't be rationally explained, so will never be resolved.

Memory 1: Bounce

The ghosts of long-gone children shriek behind the wall in the disused schoolyard at Dhuloch.

Adults can't hear these echoes—the bounce of sounds. These sounds of play are from a different time, trapped in the stones of the walls. Released, trapped again. Trapped again, released. Bounced like a ball full of grey echoes.

Only living children can hear ghost children.

'Listen to us. There's nothing there,' adults say. 'There's nothing there.'

But we are visible children so we have solid demands. We cup our hands around adults' ears, trying to open them wider, to wilder sounds.

'Listen,' we say, as we mimic the laughter of invisible children. 'There, there.'

Memory 2: Codename Trinity

I sit up in bed. My bedroom window is shut and the door is closed. I shine my torch upwards. There are five mobiles on my bedroom ceiling. Suspended from threads and wire coat hangers, hanging from white hooks.

Tin sun. Polystyrene explosion. Cardboard moon. Paper ghosts. Foil stars.

A few weeks ago, I read an illustrated book about the apocalypse called, *When the Wind Blows*.[1] I also read a poem about a *three person'd god*, 'bend your force to break, blow, burn, and make me new.'[2] Then, I read about uranium, plutonium and the first atomic bomb. Codename Trinity.

I am fifteen and my heart is already broken in three places.

I have become terrified. Of humans inventing gods. Of forceful movements. Of splitting.

The sun mobile spins and the four others are static. I point my torch at the sun. It stills.

The moon mobile spins and the four others are static. I point my torch at the moon. It stills.

Five mobiles spin one at a time. I shine light at each of them to make them stop moving.

Tin sun. Polystyrene explosion. Cardboard moon. Paper ghosts. Foil stars.

I try not to breathe too obviously. I can't sleep till the air is still.

'Please, stop breathing,' I whisper to anything that might be listening. I shine the torch beam around the room. My posters of goddesses appear and disappear. My drawings of witches. There, gone.

I switch off my torch and lie down in bed.

'OK,' I say. 'If you're a ghost, prove it. Do something.'

When I wake it's still night. There's something lying on my pillow. As limp and soft as velvet. I feel it before I see it.

A dead mouse.

I am a murderer. I kill with my demands.

I switch on my torch.

Hanging on threads from the ceiling, there are five mobiles. One of them is spinning.

Paper ghosts.

1   Raymond Briggs, *When the Wind Blows.*
2   John Donne, *Holy Sonnet XIV.*

Memory 3: Spilled Milk

White letters on a black Ouija board, an upturned glass tumbler spells:

o p e n c l o s e o p e n c l o s e o p e n c l o s e

We five teenagers each have one finger on the glass. The ghost's answer seems urgent, the glass slides fast and faster towards each letter. Repeating and repeating.

o p e n c l o s e o p e n c l o s e o p e n c l o s e

I say, 'Who asked this question—what was it?'

o p e n c l o s e o p e n c l o s e o p e n c l o s e

'I don't know.'

o p e n c l o s e o p e n c l o s e o p e n c l o s e

'Make it stop!'

o p e n c l o s e o p e n c l o s e o p e n c l o s e

The glass is too frantic.
The glass tips over and a ghost spills out.

Memory 4: The Guest

I wake. My mum stands over me. 'What's going on?' She's wearing her green velvet dressing gown and her hair's up in a towel. 'This,' she says, indicating my bed with a jerk of her head. 'What's this?'

I sit up. I'm wearing pink pyjamas and am covered in a crochet shawl. I'm lying on the wooden bed base of my single bed. A worn purple cushion functions as a pillow.

'Come with me.' She walks to my bedroom door. 'Through here.'

Gripping the shawl around me I follow her out into the corridor, around the corner and into the next room.

'There,' she says, pointing downwards. 'What's going on?'

My heavy mattress lies in a strip of sunlight on the floorboards. The purple duvet is smoothed out, the white pillow has been plumped up. A grey bedspread is folded into a square at the end of the bed.

I say, 'I must have dreamed...'

'I don't understand.'

'I must have dreamed there was someone visiting.'

We stand side by side, staring at the neatly made bed.

My mum's voice cuts through silence. 'It's so odd.'

'I don't remember,' I say. 'I can't explain.'

We strip off the bedspread, the duvet, the pillow.

'You were bloody strong in your sleep,' my mum pants as we knee and yank the mattress back to my room. 'You must have *really* wanted your invisible guest to sleep somewhere else.'

Memory 5: Gale Force

Me and my friend N are nearly eighteen. We're walking in the countryside on a windy Saturday morning. Crows bluster through clouds as we clamber over rocks and damp soil, avoiding the scratching thistles, trying to smell the gorse-flower's coconut—an exotic scent in this landscape of cow dung and nettles.

We climb a hill towards a narrow stone tower, a monument to some dead landowner. As we reach the tower we're talking about our fear of boredom. We're talking about how dim the future sometimes seems, we're talking about not really wanting to remember too much about the party last night—

I ask N, 'Do you feel lonely at parties too?'

She replies, 'Of course not. They're *parties*.'

I tell her, 'When we're out clubbing, I often drink really fast so I'm sick. Then I lock myself in the toilet cubicle and sleep on the floor till the club's about to close. I leave at the same time as everyone else.'

She frowns. 'What?'

'I don't know why,' I say. 'I know it's not the right thing to do. But it's too much, all of it. All the colours and voices and what

everyone wants is crashing like sound into all the lights and smells.
I try not to, but I kind-of have to.'
    She's about to reply—
something we can't see grips our shoulders and shoves us back
against the tower wall—
    side by side we're held firm—
    'What the hell's this?' N shrieks.
We're both trembling, spines against stone.
    I gasp, 'It's proof there's more things in the world than are visible.'
My heart wants to burst out of me and flit off into the sky.
    I gasp again. 'Feel the force of it!'
    N grips my hand, her eyes shining. 'The size of it!'
    Hope is contagious.
    We laugh and we laugh and we laugh till whatever's pinning us
down, lets go.

2016
Glass and Brick and Ice

At around midnight there is an earthquake.
7.8 magnitude felt all across central New Zealand.
I don't go outside for at least a month
because the city buildings are too tall and full of glass
or too cracked and full of brick
and because the earthquake has become trapped inside my body
like an un-solved memory.

Whenever I lie down the earthquake continues shaking
deep in my spine.
In my father's grave in Scotland
earth slowly moves around his decaying body.
His spine is a slow earthquake, shifting soil.

There's ice frozen in a protective layer
all through my heart. A crack deepens.
I only know the ice is there when I feel it shift,
an earthquake of the heart.

The Size of Love

Birds know all about love.
But you don't often understand our languages.
Shhh. Draw close. Listen.

I'm still trying to understand love.
I might never understand love.

Love is at the window.

Love is in the rain on a glass surface. In our garden in Wellington, the kōwhai tree shivers. Wind blows in circles, straining frail branches one way and the other. A pīwakawaka flits underneath the tangled rose vine and out again. The wind picks the tiny bird up by its outstretched wings, spins it and drops it over the fence, into someone else's garden. Rain blurs the windowpane, melting every shade of garden-green into vertical lines. The outside surface of the window loves rain. Water lands, pours, slides down its surface. Individual raindrops merge, group, bump, separate, bond. Glass loves rain. Rain is at this window, loving glass. I am at this window, loving rain. Love is at this window.

Love is at the door which opens for a stray ginger cat.

The hinges of our door are oiled and uncreaking so as not to scare him on his way in. The stray ginger cat knows exactly where the food and water bowls live, on our wooden floor behind this door. We call him Boy, though he might have other names. His food bowl is constantly full, in case he stops by before his usual time of after-dark. The floorboards love the touch of Boy's tiptoeing paws. The door loves these rare moments of entry and exit—the open and close, the movements of Boy's furred body or our clothed bodies passing through, shifting air. It's sometimes easier to imagine the love felt by inanimate objects and animals, rather than think about how love is experienced by humans. Especially when love became damaging in the past. Especially when someone who was much loved has died. Especially when new love coincided with the timing of that death.

Love spreads through the tissues of bodies.

In the darkest parts of the body, love cradles the most delicate organs. It grows from the heart and spreads outwards. It coils gently through the bone marrow, shifts in and out of lungs and sprackles through the skin like the electricity of sputtering lamplight. Love rises with the hair follicles. It falls away with cutaway parts: split ends, discarded skin cells and broken teeth. It causes damage when it becomes trapped in the body for too long, or is unrequited or ignored—love needs to flow through the veins, to see colour from the cones inside the eyes, it needs to feed the brain with pictures and strange ideas. Love needs to maintain interest so it can keep moving. Bodies are strong and fragile things and emotions have a bigger affect than we can understand. Kidneys can become fear-frigid, the liver can inflame with stuck-passion, the confused brain can become fog-clogged. When someone or something dies, their body becomes no more or less than a split end, a clump of fur, discarded skin cells, a trail of feathers, a broken tooth. What happens to all the love which was felt?

Love spreads through air.

It is all through the attic over our heads—the only place in this house which neither of us has ever been. There is a small trapdoor in the corridor ceiling, but the ladder is in the laundry-room under the kitchen. We used to have emergency earthquake bags down there too, until we realised that this house was the safest place to be in a real earthquake. We have not yet lived in this house for long enough to have the kinds of spare possessions that are stored in an attic. I once had a broken blue suitcase but I threw it away. I'm hoping we might never need to store anything up there and we'll always have a layer of air above us. The air in our attic secretly stores the excess of love which doesn't fit inside these rooms. It's providing an overflow area, in case we ever need to access this stockpile in love-emergencies. Air is never really an empty thing. Air loves dust, hair particles, fur and miniature things far too small for the human eye to see. It also loves vast and invisible things. It contains excess emotions—feelings too big or exuberant to be confined to human bodies. Just reach out and touch the air around someone you love. Let yourself feel how alive the air feels, let yourself feel the thickness of the air all around them, then you'll feel how big the person you love really is.

Love moves, shifts, changes shape, travels.

All the love that belonged to my once-living-loving-father, my love for him and his love for me is still here in the world. Sometimes it's trapped inside my body, sometimes it moves around me, trying to find some other place to go to. Grief is homeless love. It is love for the careful thoughts I could see in my dad's eyes, just before he cleared his throat to speak. It is love for the sound of his voice, no matter what he was saying. It is love for the way he'd solidly lay his hand across the centre of my back, so I'd feel every hug he gave me all the way through to my heart. Some of this homeless love attaches itself to other love I feel, amplifying it. The love I feel for my mum and brothers, for the stray cat Boy who habitually appears at night-time. Love for this small home which contains everything we need, for the door that locks us in safety while we sleep, for the rain that falls on one side of the windows, love for any bird who is picked up, battered and dropped by the wind. Most of all, the love I feel for Morgan that spreads throughout this house and piles up as thick clouds in the attic.

Love is painful.

Grief for my dad is worse again at the moment because I can't visit where he lived, or see any of my family for a long time. I'm full of the things I'm missing. I can't even speak about them because the missing things have piled up too high in my throat. So today I sit still, doing nothing apart from folding and unfolding my arms. It's good I'm home alone today, because there's a full moon travelling freely through the skies and it's pulling at me so hard that I'm no use to anyone. I miss seeing the open seascapes my dad knew and loved. I miss hearing the garden birds he'd fed over the years, and their chicks, and their chicks' chicks. I miss walking around the garden with him, hearing stories about the trees and shrubs he grew from seed. I miss the way he'd squeeze my hand when I cried. I miss giving my mum and brothers the best kind of hugs, because he taught me how to hug really well. I miss being hugged by him. On some days, my arms feel empty.

Love worries, frets that loved ones are in danger.

Whenever we're in the UK we can be physically close to our relatives and friends, people who have known us for a long time and enjoy seeing us together. I can watch Morgan talking intimately and laughing with her siblings. We can touch other people without worrying about crossing unfamiliar boundaries. We are invited inside other people's houses. As I look at websites which advise us not to travel *at this time*, this pandemic-time of unpredictable limits, love falls in liquid form from my eyes. I'm annoyed with myself for these private tears because in reality, *here* is brilliant. We are safe here, when so many people across the world, including our families, are not. We have made a warm loving home in this extraordinary country I'm still keen to explore, though neither of us can drive. But I also miss so much that's over there. The only cure for this kind of homesickness is to visit, but the border is closed and this impossible journey isn't safe for us, or for them. What's to be done with so much pointless *missing*? We're grounded for the foreseeable future. The Spanish Flu pandemic lasted just over two years and came in four waves. How long will this pandemic take? Who will it take? Sometimes there are no answers, only questions. These tears won't stop burning. They're full of fretful love.

Love asks difficult questions.

If love travels by air and falls inside tears, can it travel by fire and by earth as well? When my dad was dying, he gathered me, my mum and my three brothers together and asked us to discuss whether it would be 'Fire or earth?' I chose earth and neither he, nor anyone else, disagreed. I examined their eyes to be certain of this. Unflinching, my dad nodded and said, 'Burial it is, then.' His illness was already so sudden, I couldn't bear his physical body to be immediately and completely destroyed by flames. If I sit outside next to our blazing fire pit, breathe air in and out and dig my fingertips into rain-soaked earth, will I feel a deep pulse of rock through earth and know he's felt I want to visit his grave, but can't?

Love follows the things it wants.

I worry, sometimes, that my dad's ghost lingers alone next to his grave at Roucan Loch. It's a long drive from my mum's house and a long drive for each of my three brothers. It's a rural graveyard with no gravestones and young trees mark where the bodies are buried. But if he's alone and none of the other greenly buried ghosts are also wandering around, at least he'll have many varieties of tree to catalogue, and a changeable view of a big sky. Flocks of honking geese pass overhead in V-shapes. He and I used to often watch them together. I'd always point out how the leader changed from one goose to another and back again. Perhaps his ghost is hitching lifts with the geese and migrating through skies while no one else can travel. I imagine him trying out the determined wings of a goose-leader and then settling into the more relaxed wings of a follower.

Love that leads is dangerous.

To lead, to leash. A leash is attached to a collar around my neck. On the other end of the leash is a transforming person: they are a well-dressed woman, a confident man, a king, a prince, a glamorous film star, a drag queen in peacock feathers. They are multiple beautiful or delightful or popular identities—always changing but there is a yank on this collar, tight around my neck. Instead of barking, I meow. The sound wakes me up in this bed I sleep in with Morgan. Barely breathing so as not to disturb her too, I get up and gulp cold water, releasing the feeling of being held in a too-tight grip. Boy is curled on our sofa, watching me through narrowed eyes. I sit beside him for a while, listening to his purr getting louder and deeper as I gently stroke his whole spine.

Love moves even when the body is completely still.

The bedroom lamp on Morgan's side of the bed illuminates her watercolour paintings while we hold each other tight. Blues, purples, reds, greens. Whenever we're curled in each other's arms, love surrounds us. It's almost a separate thing that's wrapped around us, apart from it can't be because it's all through us as well. We've always been like this with each other. When we first fell in love from opposite sides of the world, the size and shape of love became enormous.

Love travels, moves, glows. How we think about it also changes over time. Last week I thought love and death were of equal size. But now I'm thinking love might be bigger after all. I can feel Morgan's heartbeat through my skin. It's a rhythmic beat. Definite. Confident. Taking a slow breath I think without sound, *remember this moment.* I look up at the ceiling and think of all the emergency love, stockpiled in the attic. But as I feel Morgan smile against my neck, even more love flows out of me. In this half-light, I can almost see it moving through the air over her watercolour paintings. Beside her picture of entangled dragons, a trail of blue lights. Then a flash like a miniature star over a painting of a woman in a red dress who's emerging from the sea. Half-dreaming, I close my eyes and listen to her definite, confident heartbeats.

One of us murmurs, 'I love you.' The other replies, 'Love's too small a word.'

Love can be uncontained.

Hands are designed to make things shift, grow, change, move and keep moving. Hands know how to cause pain and how to make love explode as pleasure from within the human body. People who love and are loved know how to embrace a human heart, even though it's buried deep inside the body. But in this time of being still, to keep love moving, to amplify it, direct it, follow it, or to hold it close, we don't really need our bodies at all. Just as we don't need our cutaway parts: split ends, discarded skin cells, broken teeth, all the things that fall away, eventually, the whole human body will become another cutaway part, leaving nothing but love.

Love is being in love.

When we say we are in love, we mean we are inside a place of love. We choose each other in order to stay inside and not outside this particular place of love. My mum sends me a photograph of the smokebush outside her back door. Rain glistens like enormous tears on blood red leaves. The plant looks familiar and alive, but it's so far away from this place of love I've chosen to be inside.

The moon pulls at me again as it circles around the world. Morgan and I used to write to each other about the moon when we were first falling in love. The moon rose and fell in our different hemispheres, linking us together. I sent the full moon to Morgan wearing a scarf made of flies. She sent me a half-moon with bruises on her face. I sent her a cloud-bound moon, surrounded by the stars who had taken her hostage. There were many moons. My favourite moon was one of Morgan's—a moon who was being hunted by a great wolf and this dark moon wanted the wolf to catch and eat her, because she was deep-sick in love with the wolf.

Love is airborne.

Love moves in through opening-closing windows and flows out through opening-closing doors. It repeats itself as a word too small for its meanings. It is tiptoed on by stray cats. It rises into the attics of happy homes. It moves through the wind, shifting small birds from one garden into another. It ruffles the leaves of the kōwhai tree. It travels on slow breath, reminding us—keep feeling. It follows migrations of birds which make V-shapes through the sky. Morgan and I are often homesick but we live inside a place of love, still telling each other stories about the moon. And while we're not even noticing it, love moves invisibly around our bodies, never quite letting us see that we are far bigger than we appear.

Kōwhai Tree

I wish I could transform   new things
into old friends   just by looking at them   for long enough.
There's the black-green   feathers of a Tūī   as it drinks desperate nectar -
its voice is a bell   a crack   a telephone's ring.
It's the kind of bird who chases away anything that looks the same as itself.
Morning dreams of missing faces talking   missing years   missing voices
A crowd   of hers and hims and theys and shes and hes and thems and yous.
I'm sleep-listening without hearing   because everyone I miss   talks all at once.
Thought paths like disappearing plane-trails   is this too far to write lines to?
Everyone ignores   migration   sees   only what   is exactly *here*.
So I'm sending   invisible airmail   in pictures and noise—
have this glimpse—   light   such soft   yellow flowers
and the sound   of three clocks ticking   through another quiet day.
If you look, I'll show you this   Kōwhai tree, flowering—
between brown seeds   in hanging   vertical gulps.
The grip of Tūī-claws   make petals   shake and fall   sipping nectar
on branches   they don't even scratch. I'll show you the daffodils I didn't
know grew here   tall in a vase. The sunshine from the window reflects
in my lover's blue-blue eyes.   She loves this country
I'm thumb-printing   condensation   gradients:
glass-widths   dream-depths,   some map I once travelled   cold.
here, there's love   and the real things   I can hold
in both eyes   the sound of   envelopes   torn open.
A bird   in a tree.   Spring.
Soon there will be
a birthday
where I'll
remember
people who
know me.
Remember
having
friends
close
enough
to party
with,
but
for
now
there's
this
kiss.

Weather Bomb

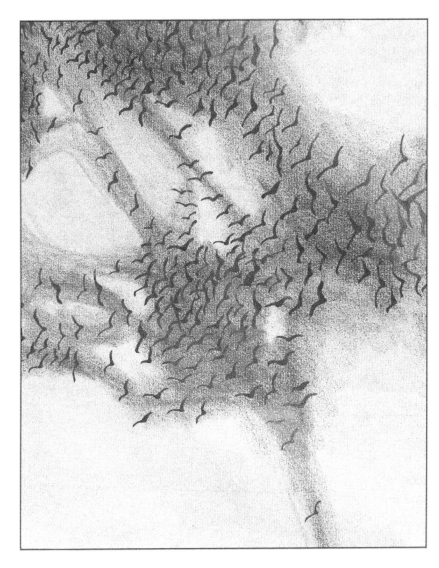

Vortex II

Six Words for Loneliness

Despane– The loneliness of feeling misunderstood, unloved or unheard by someone who used to understand, love or listen.

Starn– Craving something or someone to be there but knowing it's/ they're not. Wanting to bite something.

Youache– Where a specific person is missed and only their physical presence will cure the ache of missing them.

Ignornly– The kind of loneliness that other people notice, but don't mention to the person they think is lonely. Their expression shows sympathy, but also a little wariness, as if loneliness could be contagious.

Solilone– A type of melancholia experienced while gazing at a wide-skied landscape. A longing for strangeness, for the unreal or the surreal to appear.

Idealone– A hankering for an imagined scenario—where it's the idea of the situation that causes the loneliness. For example, the 'ideal' of the perfect friend sitting opposite on the sofa, laughing over wine and confessions and saying all of the right things.

Small Talk

My first work party in New Zealand is on a floor in the High School I don't usually go to. I'm late and a bit lost.

Rush.

Damp-smelling corridors, rows of lockers.

The scent of some green soap that doesn't exist anymore. A corner.

Posters of poems on the walls.

Double doors.

Squares of frosted glass, the colours move as liquid, distorted shapes.

The party is a piece of sensory abstract art. Blue, aqua. Green, white.

I reach out my fingertips, to touch the party from outside.

Footsteps from behind me, interrupt.

Open the doors and walk through.

Inside the party:

paper chains

fifty people gathered in small groups.

Empty chairs around coffee tables.

The office administrators, L and K, provide drinks from behind a hatch. I wave hello as I pick up a plastic cup of orange juice. L beams at me as she uses both her hands and one of K's to fill a row of precarious cups from an oversized bottle of white wine. 'Hey Jess, you well?'

'Fine thanks—I thought you'd be partying too, not sorting the drinks out?'

K shrugs. 'We'll join in later.'

It's a shame they're locked away behind another hatch—much like the office hatch they work behind on the floor below this one.

Though I only work here for two hours a week, as I arrive or depart they are often talking about blustery things:

technology dysfunction,

embarrassing relatives
too-late too-rude emails
early bad-weather
irrational complaints
unforgivable new rules.
But they're not talking, tonight.

Clasping my orange juice I stand near the food table. If anyone else arrives knowing no one, they'll hover here too. They might talk to me.

New arrivals scan the table for unspillable foods.

A tall man in thick glasses asks me, 'What do you teach?'

'Creative writing.' I reply, trying to make eye contact. 'I teach it here in the evenings and part time at the University, on and off. And you?'

'Marketing,' he says, examining a plate of dips.

I've heard of marketing, but don't quite know what it is.

I ask, 'What do you like best about it?'

My small-talk small-voice isn't big enough.

He spikes two chunks of pale cheese onto a stick, waves at a cluster of grey-suited tutor, and strides away.

I half-respect him for not even pretending to be nice.

I've been inside this party for five and a half minutes.

Sipping my juice I feel like a child and regret not choosing wine.

The second hand moves around the clock.

There are many bright patterns and textures of clothing. Music is playing but I can't tell what the tune is.

People's smiles are facial punctuation, the comma while the mouths prepare their next phrase.

Someone walks past me.

There's a smell of floral perfume and wine and antiseptic wipes.

Another someone walks past in the opposite direction.

Cheese and onion crisps, nailpolish remover and strawberries.

I'm going to allow myself to leave after I've been inside this party for a total of fifteen minutes, unless someone I look at speaks to me. Then I have to stay till the conversation is over.

Two ladies with dark hair and wine in plastic cups sit in the chairs next to me.

They look like they might have come to New Zealand from another country too, which immediately gives me a whole range of questions to ask them. But the one closest to me turns her chair away so they're facing each other. The back of her long hair is clenched in a delicate butterfly clip.

One says to the other, 'Lovely to catch up with you!'

'You too! It's been ages since we last talked. In the staffroom, wasn't it?'

'Weeks! How's crochet class going?'

One of their voices sounds happy, but the other is only pretending to be happy.

A lot of adults feel extreme emotions inside schools. Memories are locked in the old smells which linger in the walls. The two dark-haired ladies whisper about a couple, hand in hand.

'Partners aren't allowed. It was clear on the invite.'

'Maybe they're both tutors.'

'How funny.'

I've been inside this party for exactly fifteen minutes.

I put my empty cup and plate in the recycling bins.

By the doors there's a leaving card.

Pausing, I write, *Sorry you're leaving, K. You've been lovely to say hello to each week.*

I hope you get to enjoy a proper party soon, where someone else pours drinks for you. Jx

So, I'm rubbish at small-talk. Why can't I learn how to do it better so it keeps going till it turns into big-talk?

I was probably never designed to be an ease-myself-in kind of immigrant. But then again, maybe no one is ever really designed to leave or arrive anywhere at all. I imagine immigrants who find it easy are extroverts, or have strong faith in the concept of settling-in.

Didn't the Greek gods blow ships around, just for the chaos of moving people from one piece of land to another?

But whatever forces cause us to move, we all either leave or arrive somewhere, or stay in the same haunted place.

Walking home I replay each moment of the party over and over again, watching what happens.

Then I replay each moment over and over again, trying to change what happened.

I imagine the evening went like this:

The man with thick glasses doesn't disappear, so I ask him to tell me how interesting marketing is for him. He takes me over to the whiteboard and hands me a black pen. He explains that marketing is a secretive area of study, concerned primarily with the sale of miniature items within miniature markets. Miniature markets only sell miniature magical things, like very small singing cats or levitating toothpicks or talking teaspoons or flying grapes or leaping caterpillars or flammable ice cubes. The man in thick glasses continues to talk while I fill the whiteboard with intricate drawings of the miniature magical objects at each miniature market. Everyone at the party thinks we've all got such rapport, we must have known each other for ages. Soon everyone is merrily drunk and singing songs about miniature cats.

The two ladies with dark hair remove their hair clips and it falls down their backs in beautiful coils. I move my chair closer to theirs so I can ask them where they've come from. It turns out that like me, they've travelled across many skies and oceans to arrive here in New Zealand. They tell me they came here to see the long white clouds. As they begin to tell me the fascinating stories of their travels, I realise that their mouths aren't moving. Their stories are being told by their hair and each coil has its own voice. I am mesmerised by the stories in their hair, as more and more stories are told simultaneously, it's like being inside some strange hair-dream of spinning and blowing, twisting and dancing. When the hair tales have all been told, the two ladies ask me to plait their hair together, so they will never be parted. Their plait of hair whispers to itself for hours. At the end of the evening, the two women have fallen in love and decided to set up home together. They are grateful to me for bonding them together so well. We swear to each other we will always be friends.

2019
Long White Clouds

Ask any kid in an A-line skirt and long socks
to whisper their story. They'll show you the stars and their scars,
all the way from Z to aye. Far more than is visible.

Curiosity lives in the cracks in these walls,
in the eyes of hidden rats,
the splits in the pavements, jagged lines in tarred roads.
Earth splits and shakes wherever new life can shoot.

It's the familiar birds who shouldn't be here
that call clouds into the heart, singing of
a bone-deep homesickness.

So quiet. Sharp-beaked, pecking at shadows.

Dhuloch

Up till I left home at seventeen, my family lived in Dhuloch Schoolhouse—a house with an adjoining derelict school. Dhu-loch translates to Black Lake. It was an isolated stone building on a small hill. It stood among farmed fields on a remote peninsula in south west Scotland. Gale force winds. Jagged coastline.

The black loch which the school was named after was at the bottom of the hill—but not all the time. The loch only appeared when it rained.

The schoolhouse was fairly conventional—a fire in the living room, a kitchen with a four-ring cooker. Upstairs, three small bedrooms and a leaky bathroom. Most things were in need of some kind of care, or repair. While we four children were still young enough to share bunkbeds, we all lived in this damp schoolhouse. It had housed a succession of head-teachers and their families, before us.

The derelict school next door was far more interesting.

The school had stone walls, thick enough to contain secret passageways. The high ceilings were cracked and the plaster was broken in places, but they also had square, oblong, circular trapdoors leading to out-of-reach attics. Wooden cladding spanned the bottom half of the internal walls. There were rows of rusted cloakroom hooks, cracked ceramic basins, hinged desks with empty inkwells.

A square window, high in an internal wall was designed for a teacher to have a hawks-eye view over two classrooms at once. Boxes and crates and objects from the local museum were being 'kept in storage' in the classrooms. To us children the most interesting stored exhibits were the crate full of hip bones and skulls, the agricultural tools and a wooden boat so stained it must have been dug up from underground.

Layers of paint peeled from the classroom walls. Psychiatric green overlaid with white. Web-threads and plaster dust descended from exposed wooden beams. The window panes were cracked. There were tin buckets, plastic tubs, bowls, a trough placed around the floors to catch rain. A massive key shed crumbs of rust when it turned in the front door lock.

At different times of the year, the remains of trapped things appeared. Dead flies. Dead birds. Dead butterflies.

The school was haunted, of course. How could it not be? It was Victorian and full of echoes. Outside, in the overgrown playground, there were often the sounds of children playing behind a wall. When we siblings went to look for them, they'd gone.

Inside the school, there was one particular ghost I was terrified of. I'm still scared as I remember it now. This is a distant memory— in terms of time as well as location. And yet I have to talk myself into being able to mention it.

Reasons it's probably safe to mention the ghost:

a) Because of the pandemic I'm unlikely to be able to go back there any time soon.

b) It's a Scottish ghost, so it can't hear me from here in New Zealand.

c) Any previous connection between me and this ghost must, by now, be fully severed. Like a tether or a divorce.

d) This particular ghost has a very peculiar smell so I would recognise it anywhere.

e) I have never smelled the ghost anywhere but in Dhuloch School.

When I was ten, my parents got a mortgage. The museum removed the stored boxes, crates, artefacts, collections. My parents, wielding sledgehammers, knocked a door-shaped hole in the adjoining wall between the schoolhouse and the school.

Timber frames were constructed within the first classroom to build two plasterboard bedrooms and a shower.

My older brother and I moved into the school through the hole in the wall.

The smell of the ghost would appear in one of the classrooms at dusk. The texture of the smell was thicker than the scents of decay, the tone of it was darker than blood or sulphur. The sound of the smell was a bass drone in a minor key. The smell had substance; it thickened the air.

The feeling of something large. Something dangerous—the feeling of something angry.

Everyone could smell it. This ghost didn't discriminate. It wanted all of us to know it was there.

My mum described the smell as mealy. I described it as the smell of something dead. My dad would wrinkle up his whole face and say nothing. My brothers would smell it then immediately go elsewhere to avoid it.

When our parents' friends visited, they'd comment on its oddness and ask if we'd looked everywhere, for anything rotten. But the strangest thing of all was that it wasn't constant. Like the black loch we watched for from the many-paned windows, the smell came and went.

My dad and J the builder made a trapdoor in the wooden floor of one of the classrooms. They dressed in rough clothes and thick gloves. They went through the trapdoor into the three-foot gap between the floorboards and soil. They were looking for dead rats, broken drains, dead cats, overflowing sewage, dead mice.

My mum and I stood on the dusty floorboards listening to their silence beneath our feet.

I whispered, 'What do you think they're seeing?'

She replied, 'They're very quiet.'

I imagined them finding undead Victorian teachers. Being caught in a swarm of over-agitated Victorian children. I visualised my dad and J coming out of the trapdoor, destroyed by fear. Speechless. Tongueless. White as seafoam.

Lying face down, I shuffled forwards and peered beneath the floorboards. There was no daylight in that void between floor and soil.

My mum's voice. 'What're they doing?'

'They're still looking.'

The stretched shadows of two hunched men shone torches through darkness, searching for something they never found.

I watched them, trying to see a ghost in their torchlight. But it's impossible to see something which hides when light touches it.

I often couldn't sleep, knowing the ghost was only a plasterboard wall-width away from my bed. Sometimes it was inside my bedroom, spinning the mobiles on my ceiling one by one. Sometimes I thought it wanted to slip into me and wear me like a cloak. It moved small objects, often placing them in the centre of my circular rug. A bottle lid. A razor. A matchbox.

As I lay in bed with my eyes closed, the air around me prickled as if millions of tiny needles were pointing at my skin. I was made of skin cells, all vibrating—*go away. Stay quiet. Stay still...*

When I was a teenager, I wanted to understand what we were living with. My friends and I set up camp in one of the classrooms and assembled a Ouija board to try to talk to the ghost. As the glass spelled answers to our questions across the lettered board I learned that the ghost hated the words *dead, death, passed, crossed over, elapsed, deceased, expired, died.* If any of these words were spoken, the ghost became incomprehensibly angry—talking in a rush of letters with no combined meaning.

Tipping the glass as if freeing itself, we'd all feel its uncontained rage swirling beside us, through us, all around the classroom.

After a while, the Ouija board sessions ended up being more about what the living wanted to say to each other, but couldn't say aloud. Each finger placed gently on a glass could push without seeming to push, could accuse without consequence. I stopped using the Ouija board as a method of communication when I noticed a couple of my friends had realised they could make the ghost *appear* to talk.

When I saw whose eyes were seeking out letters in advance and weren't fixed on the moving glass, I understood where the power really lay.

It's strange, thinking about these memories now. From here in a kitchen in Wellington, on an October afternoon. In Scotland, it's night time and the clocks have just gone back an hour. Winter approaches. Here, sunshine and a cold breeze are coming in through the open windows. Hay fever is an itch in my skin. There's no one here to remember with me, to tell me, *yes, I remember. It was really frightening.* Or to tell me, *no, there was no ghost—it was all a weird tangle in your teenage head.*

I'm so unsettled by these memories that I'm trying to hold onto solid, ordinary things. I've potted some young tomato plants. Done our laundry on a sunny-windy day. Hugged Morgan while she was still half-asleep. Made dippy eggs for her when she was sad. Remembered to send an air mail card at least three weeks in advance of my middle brother's birthday. I've been stood here by the sofa with Morgan, watching the news, wondering when we might see our families again. I've also checked my emails, bank balance, and opened and closed the metal letterbox which a spider lives in, on our gate.

I'm working from home—preparing future-classes, marking assignments. There's a more permanent job that looks interesting but I'm not applying because it's based in Christchurch. Morgan's been there a few times and thinks that Christchurch is very haunted.

Wellington isn't haunted. It might have individual haunted houses, or it might not. I've been inside very few people's homes. This might be a cultural difference between New Zealand and the UK—being invited inside people's homes to get to know them. Or it might be that I'm still too new here, or too quiet, or too odd (and therefore suspicious). There's a superstition in the UK that if there's a knock on your door but when you open it no-one's there, you must never say *come in*. If you do, you'll be welcoming in a vampire or a witch or a ghost. Maybe there's something of that same superstition here too. I'm too invisible to be invited in. Or it might simply be that people only want to see long-term friends and relatives during a global pandemic.

I don't want to know which one of these things it is.

When we two older siblings left home for college and university, our parents and two younger brothers moved into the school through the hole in the wall.

My parents bricked the hole up again, behind them.

The schoolhouse was put on the market to be sold.

Just before the schoolhouse was handed over to the buyers, my mum rang me from their kitchen in the school and said, 'The ghost's moved next door.'

I said, 'Your new neighbours might not last long, then.'

She laughed. 'You never know, they might be down to earth. Or oblivious. More able to blank it out.'

'Why are you so sure the ghost's moved?'

She replied, 'When I went back in to air the rooms, I could smell it in the kitchen. Did you ever smell it in the schoolhouse, anywhere?'

'No, never. I felt something threatening occasionally, but never a smell. It must have been a different one.'

'Ah well. Good luck to them and however many ghosts they've ended up with.'

I laughed. 'Maybe they'll be religious and can get a priest to flick some holy water around.'

She replied, 'I'll suggest it, if they come round asking.'

My parents converted derelict Dhuloch School into their home. It took many years and bank loan after bank loan. They built a kitchen in half of a classroom and a sitting room in the other half. They re-tiled the roof. They cleaned and damp-proofed and filled and sanded and wallpapered. Blank walls were coloured-in with yellow ochre. Terracotta. Dark blue. They glued up patterned wallpapers bought from Glasgow in the January sales. They lowered some of the ceilings for warmth, making reachable attics beneath unreachable attics. One of the classroom ceilings was left at its original height. It was too high to clean without hiring scaffold towers, so once it was repaired and painted dusty pink, no one ever did.

Across the ceiling of this classroom, spiders built an inverted city—nests linked by layers of threads and passageways, woven domes and tunnels. The spiders bred ruthlessly over the years. They ate each other's babies and tore the heads off their lovers up in their city on the ceiling. There must be thousands of them by now, living out their passionate and deadly dramas.

Each summer in that classroom, hundreds of cluster flies die on the windowsills. The spiders eye the flies from above, ignoring their own hunger. Their silk threads are reserved for architectural repairs. For new developments. For spire and walkway assemblage.

My dad was protective of the spiders and their right to a home. Though when he died my mum threw out many of the things he'd been hoarding, she and the spiders still live there together. The spiders live above, she and her two tabby cats below.

Both sets of inhabitants gradually construct, deconstruct, and reconstruct their homes.

Dhuloch School is surrounded by a garden filled with hundreds of birds. There are blackbirds, chaffinches, pigeons. Every few days my mum fills about fifteen bird feeders with different kinds of seeds. There are greenfinches, blue tits, goldfinches. She piles stale breadcrumbs on the stone tables in the garden which my dad somehow built while no one was looking. There are swifts, robins, swallows. There are kestrels, gulls, and occasionally a heron. There's a constant sound of birdsong from dawn till dusk. There are crows, rooks, pheasants. From dusk back to dawn there are the night-calls of owls.

I miss Dhuloch School, as the home it was for my parents, as the home it has become for my mum. I miss it because it contains my family's memories. I miss it because it still contains objects my dad touched.

I'm trying to plant my feet more firmly on the ground. Right here. Duppa Street, Wellington. Our tomato plants are growing bigger alongside each other, outside in the garden. I'm in the kitchen. Morgan's editing the proofs for her debut novel in the front room. We've been quiet all day and have barely spoken at all. We speak in the language of small touches, my hand to her shoulder, her forehead to my lips.

The tūī and blackbirds and sparrows are clicking and clacking and trilling their songs in the neighbours' enormous tree. The house beneath the tree is now empty because the couple who rented it have moved away, to be nearer their families in Christchurch.

I don't like being next door to an empty house.

But in a global pandemic, it appears that most people want to be nearer their families.

Nearer to places containing memories.

Nearer to the past, because the future is so uncertain.

Even when the past is a haunted place.

Pretending to be Rain

I'm employed to teach on short-term contracts at one of the local universities. I consider myself lucky to have any job at all as they're not easy to find. Since the pandemic began, they're also not easy to keep. Today, I'm on campus at an annual meeting. After watching three important people speaking for nearly two hours about nothing that's fixed itself in my mind, there's a coffee break.

Everyone gathers in a room that smells of new carpets.

Two of the academic staff I've spoken to on and off during the past year are beside me at the refreshments table. I and H are full-time academics and are friends with each other outside work. H lives within walking distance of Berhampore. He often walks his dog along our road, though he's never seen me looking out through the front window. I lives nearer the university campus.

They're talking about a novel they've recently discussed in their book group.

I'm pouring hot water onto coffee grains as I say, 'A book group must be fun.'

I frowns at the large plate of chocolate biscuits. 'Not dairy-free.' She wanders off towards the fridge.

I say to H, 'Does the group meet in your home?'

'It's very academic.' He sniffs the milk jug.

My stomach growls because I forgot to eat breakfast. Taking two biscuits I say, 'That sounds interesting.'

He removes his string-dangling tea bag and bumps drips from it, once, twice. '*Very* academic,' he repeats, dropping the teabag in a small tabletop bin. He nods at the biscuits in my hand. 'You'd think they'd at least get a cake, or something containing moisture.'

He smiles at me sideways, pretending something I can't recognise.

Crossing the room, he joins I on a red sofa.

They glance at me, clearly checking I'm not going to be joining them.

Frowning, I turn towards a window looking out on a small square between university buildings. I've got a PhD but I'm not academic enough. A small lawn. Paving stones. I've published three novels, but I'm not clever enough to discuss books. Herbs and native shrubs.

Maybe they just don't want me to come into their houses.

I wonder why not. My eyes sting. I'm too sensitive.

I've always been too sensitive.

It's humid today. I find a metal lever and open the window. It won't extend more than a crack. The scents of smoky flax plants and calming lavender come in, competing.

I place my coffee on the windowsill. With my back to the room, I dunk my biscuits and while eating them, a seagull lands on the grass outside.

The seagull looks amazingly white.

It glows as it hops, shuffles, stamps.

Whatever was really just being said in that odd conversation is probably much bigger in my head than it should be. Like imagining a storm when it's only spitting with rain. But recently I've become very unsure about how to choose people to talk to. How do I pick people who'll talk about things they're passionately interested in? How can I tell by looking at people, which one might listen to my interests? I glance around the room at all the academics who are talking or not talking, in groups or alone, examining their phones, trying not to think about how soon they have to go back into the meeting.

Even in my late forties I am still an odd girl who doesn't understand anything about anyone. I'm only here because I got a vague group message saying this meeting presented a rare opportunity for staff 'at all levels' to network. I can see the levels, the hierarchy, and I know exactly where I am within it. But I'm uncomfortable in groups, so don't understand what networking really means. Perhaps only spiders or crochet teachers are good at this—seeing the net and all its strands from within. Seeing how to work a route out of it, how to find a way from one vantage point to another. How to find the most useful people and convince them they're not being...used.

I shouldn't have come. I can never see anything I'm neck-deep in. I'm blind to it, while inside. What else am I blind to, that I'm right in the middle of?

Everyone's pretending coffee-time is eternal, because the second half of the meeting is going to be duller than the first. Because most people in this room are permanent staff who have never met someone as temporary as me, I'll be too visible if I walk the straight line from this window to the door and leave now. I wish G was here, but she's not in today. She helped me to get this temporary job after we first met on a writing panel. She works from home a lot and lives further up the coast, with chickens. G's not from New Zealand either, though she's lived here twenty years or more. I want to be at home with Morgan. I came to New Zealand for her, for love. But here I am, also trying to do something else. Earn money. Begin to think about the future again? Make friends. Communicate in ways that I must have once thought were easy or ordinary. When was that? There's no good reason to be here in this group of people, not really. There are about a million good reasons to go back home to Morgan.

I'll wait till they all return to the meeting and slip away.

Leaning against the windowsill, I try to work out whether the crumbs at the bottom of my coffee cup will float if I gently swirl it around.

Many years ago I worked as a chambermaid and didn't have to talk to anyone apart from the hotel receptionist, who I collected the bundle of room keys from. I could imagine all kinds of stories while cleaning up after transient people. I could think whatever I wanted while I scrubbed and polished and wiped and smoothed, because they weren't paying me for my thoughts.

This room is full of people who are paid to think. All of their thoughts are loud, some chant, some flutter, some bellow, some stomp. All of the thoughts in this room are talking at the same time as each other, though the people who are thinking them aren't all speaking.

The air between the tops of our heads and the ceiling tiles is thick and I can't look directly at it in case I start seeing their thoughts as storm clouds or thread-words. Is it all the things we learn which made our thoughts louder, or do thoughts become loud because there's an unfulfilled desire—the need to be heard?

Turning back to the window, I watch the glowing seagull. It yellow-eyes the ground with black-rimmed intensity and resumes stamping. My foot taps along a little and makes me smile.

The seagull is pretending to be rain.

It's trying to trick earthworms into rising to the surface so it can grab them and slurp them into its beak. Will the worms die inside the gull's beak, or neck, or guts? Does one place cause a more painful death, than another? I imagine worms might feel more surprised about this kind of death, rather than fearful. I wait for the seagull's beak to prod, jab the ground. Behind me, the room grows quieter as it gradually empties.

Outside, it starts to rain. Now the earthworms must have conflicting ideas about which part of the soil to rise through.

The seagull loses interest and flies off.

Maybe earthworms aren't blind to the soil they're in, or the danger they're beneath. They feel what's around them by using senses other than sight. Textures and movement, vibrations and sounds must fill the soil they writhe through. They feel for water, sensing rain.

As I leave the university building and walk home,
   I pretend to be rain.
    I am blinding rain and I am blind as rain.
     I am a clattering timpani sound.
      I am a running, pooling, dripping thing.
       Drenching the roofs and gutters
      Clearing the underground pipes of debris I
     roll downwards, away.
   Soaking the walls of every building in this city
I splatter and splutter across all the washing left hanging on lines.
Drip-dancing in puddles
  sliding down all the front doors
    I'm rain,
      falling against one side of the windows.
                I'm outside.

Weather Bomb

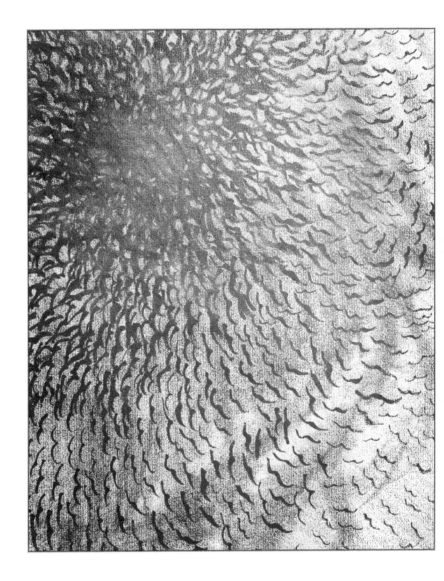

Vortex III

Seven Words for Loneliness

Despane– The loneliness of feeling misunderstood, unloved or unheard by someone who used to understand, love or listen.

Starn– Craving something or someone to be there but knowing it's/ they're not. Wanting to bite something.

Youache– Where a specific person is missed and only their physical presence will cure the ache of missing them.

Ignornly– The kind of loneliness that other people notice, but don't mention to the person they think is lonely. Their expression shows sympathy, but also a little wariness, as if loneliness could be contagious.

Solilone– A type of melancholia experienced while gazing at a wide-skied landscape. A longing for strangeness, for the unreal or the surreal to appear.

Idealone– A hankering for an imagined scenario—where it's the idea of the situation that causes the loneliness. For example, the 'ideal' of the perfect friend sitting opposite on the sofa, laughing over wine and confessions and saying all of the right things.

Achiposs– The ache of missing out on experiencing something beautiful, because it is impossible.

Doves

In this memory, I'm around twenty and sleep-deprived. I've arrived at my parents' house after an eighteen-hour train journey. It's about one in the morning and my younger brothers are asleep. My parents sit opposite me at the kitchen table where I'm eating thick broccoli soup. I tell them about a woman I didn't meet at one of the stations I got stranded at on the way here.

'*Didn't* meet?' says my dad.

'Didn't meet.' I reply.

She was talking to someone else and I was on my own, waiting for a delayed train connection. All the Victorian fixtures at the station were painted green and red. Somewhere between a remote place in Devon and a remote place in Scotland. Maybe Preston. I often get stuck at Preston. I tell my parents, 'I completely recognised her, even though I don't know her and have never met her before.'

My mum asks me to describe her.

So, I tell them about her heart-shaped face, her brilliant-blue eyes, her long grey hair, metal bangles and the tiny bells on her lilac scarf. I tell them I could hear her soulful voice singing in my head. She was a few feet away from me, quietly listening and laughing with her friend.

'I know her.' I say. 'But I don't. And she knows me. But she doesn't.' I get up from the table and go over to the sink to rinse out my bowl.

'Did you talk to each other?' My dad asks.

Still running the tap, I shake my head. 'We don't, do we. Talk to strangers with no tangible reason. I wasn't even meant to be there in that moment, in Preston or wherever. I was meant to be four hours further north. So. Her friend is talking and me and her, well we keep glancing at each other. She's the sound of bells. She's a dove crossed with an angel crossed with sea foam.'

My mum looks me up and down, taking in my dyed-black hair, long black coat, Stripy red and black tights. Army surplus boots. I'm quiet for a moment, thinking about bright colours hidden underneath white lace curtains...

My mum says, 'You look as dark as she was light.'

Reaching for the kettle, I ask, 'Do you want tea as well?'

My dad shakes his head. 'We'll head to bed as soon as you're sorted out. And then what?'

I turn on the kettle. 'So, my delayed train arrives and I get on it. But I don't sit down yet. I turn and face the window. And I'm stood at the window, still looking at her, as the whistle shrieks and the train starts to move. She sees me. *Really* sees me. Leaving her friend mid-sentence, gaping after her, she strides across the platform towards my train. She touches one side of the window with the whole palm of her hand and I touch the other as the train picks up speed. Our hands touch without touching through a layer of glass and both our eyes are full of tears. I can hear the sound of a bell clanging. We're smiling at each other as she walks along beside the train, then as she runs we're laughing and almost crying at the same time. And then...'

I take a deep breath. 'And then she's gone. I'm gone. As if neither of us were ever there at all.'

My throat feels tight as I search the cupboards for a chamomile teabag and my favourite patterned mug. I say, 'And I know her but don't know her. I've met her over and over again, but never met her.'

They glance at each other and my dad says, 'Reincarnation. You must have known each other in another life.' My mum takes his hand and he strokes her fingers.

I pour water on the teabag. My eyes fill with tears because I miss her so much, this woman I didn't meet today. I say, 'Maybe. But what's the point in reincarnation, if we recognise each other but can't remember why? It's like a recycling mistake.'

My mum rests her head on my dad's shoulder and it makes me smile, seeing them like this.

'I'll let you get to bed.' I scoop up my kit bag and sling it over my shoulder. Picking up my steaming mug I say, 'Wrong lifetime or wrong place or wrong face. Wrong species, maybe.' I go towards the door.

Pausing, I turn back to face them. 'Christians might say she was an angel. But angels have purpose, don't they? There are reasons for them being there, all pale and beautiful and lace-like and feathered, reasons which are quickly revealed? Is reincarnation this cruel, to have no reasons? She was a dove. Sea foam. A...' A tear leaks down my face.

'You're overtired.' my mum says, getting up from the table and putting her hand on my shoulder. 'Do you remember when you were really little—you told me we'd been here before. And you said that in the before-time, it was the other way around. You were big and I was small?'

I nod. 'I half-remember it. But more than whatever it was we said, I remember feeling worried about your feet.'

She looks at my dad with a smile that tells me they've already had this conversation.

He has a knowing tone in his voice as he says, 'China. Foot binding.'

'Maybe.' I say. 'I've always wanted to go there, but never known quite why. How long does it take, after death. For a dead person to be recycled into another body, do you think? When would the woman on the train station have died? When would I have died?'

My dad smiles at my mum.

Her hand rests gently on my shoulder.

My dad gets up, saying, 'Bed now.'

Frowning, I say, 'I daydreamed through too much science at school. Is time definitely linear?'

Both of them laugh at me. 'Bed! Get some rest.'

'Glad you're finally here.' My dad puts his arm around me and strokes my back.

I grin at him. 'Me too. Thanks for staying up. I'm sorry I'm this late.'

I always talk too much the first night I arrive here. Partly because the journey is so long and I always think a lot while moving from one place to another. And partly because they pay attention to what I'm saying before we settle into the good and bad habits we have when we're around each other. By tomorrow evening we'll all have slipped into only half-listening, or being annoying, or bickering, or being carelessly occupied with other things. But the arrival nights are special. It's always late, so it's usually just me and them together. I feel like they really see me because they're looking for what's changed in me since leaving home, looking for what stays the same.

To me, they are always the same. Believing in astrology, tarot, reincarnation, runes and all kinds of odd healing practices, as if these are the easiest and most natural things to believe in. They are the same whenever I visit. Yes, sometimes one talks more than the other, sometimes they are angry or fearful, hopeful or fretful or joyful. But underneath however they appear, they are each of them fixed in place as themselves. Their house is full of books and pictures and pets and musical instruments and colours. It's them and my brothers I come all this way to see, not ex-school friends or ex-work colleagues, ex-teachers, and not the place.

I still don't know what I believe in. A few weeks ago I believed in a Goddess who had the head of a cat. I used to know a boy who believed in a brick and I could see that for him, the brick, at least, was reliable. When I was fifteen I believed my bedroom was possessed by an angry teenage ghost. A couple of months ago I was convinced we were all *inside* something so vast, we couldn't see what it was. As if the planet earth was a tiny piece of dust inside an elephant's gallbladder. Recently I've been wondering if all humans are different kinds of animals, insects and birds, in disguise. And the purpose of this 'human disguise'? It's designed to make us believe we are united at the top of the food chain, so we don't eat each other. But our true natures still show through.

I kiss my mum (a disguised crow) and my dad (a disguised badger) good night. Switching the corridor light on, I tiptoe along the wooden floorboards trying not to wake my younger brothers or spill my tea. In the spare bedroom there's the smell of dusty books. I drop my bag on the floor and sit on the single bed. It's covered with a patchwork blanket. The bedside lamp is angled. It shines a circle of light on the dark blue wall, where they've hung a framed watercolour picture I did while I was at secondary school.

In the picture, a solitary witch examines darkness flowing from her hands. Her hair, the river, the clouds and a thin tree fill the painting all around her with swirls, containing or trapping her inside the image. The darkness is coming from within her, threatening to spread like a vortex and consume everything around her—the indigo water, the ink-lines of thin air, the burnt umber branches of the tree—all these things the witch once loved so much. I was sad when I painted this picture. My best friend had become very religious.

Her religion forbade her to be friends with me, so she stopped. I didn't know how to get her to come back to me again because her religion was a dream I couldn't wake her from. At some point her family moved away. She was light as well. Light and blonde. Pale as a dove. Gone.

She wasn't the woman at the train station but like her, she'd seemed familiar when I first met her. I miss her in the same way as I now miss the woman at the train station.

Perhaps there are many doves in our lives, all around us, but just passing through. They're not meant to be kept, to be known. They are meant to be longed for. They don't want any memories or darkness or depth to be attached to them.

They want to be remembered as something beautiful that almost-was.

As a something which is a nothing.

As a nothing that is light

fleeting

gone.

Headless Ghost

Tonight, Boy goes outside through the cat flap. On the kitchen table, I'm drawing in pencil and ink—a picture of a flock of birds. Boy thumps and bumps outside on the deck. He's playing with something in the darkness. Through the glass doors I catch the odd flash of his ginger fur. Ears, flicking tail. Paws.

Moth-catching.

Sometimes I forget he's a wild animal. Out there in the world of nocturnal creatures, everything eats everything else.

He miaows at the cat flap to be let back in again. We keep the catch on exit-only because the neighbour's hungry cat is on a special diet.

As I unbolt and open the glass door, Boy comes in, making a miaow that sounds like he's curling his teeth around an off-key musical note.

'What is it, Boy?'

'Mrouow.'

'Come on, then.' I close and bolt the door.

'Mrououw.' He looks up at me insistently.

'You've had food. And water. It's still there, look.' I gesture at the bowls on the floorboards.

'Mrouwow.'

'I don't know what you want.'

Morgan's watching the news. She calls from the sofa, 'He wants your attention.'

I stroke him and he nudges his head against my shin. A few moments later he goes outside again, thudding through the cat flap.

Picking up a brush pen, I draw bird shapes across a pencil cloud. The birds multiply, spreading wing lines across this sheet of textured white paper.

On the news, the reporter is talking about a new strain of the Covid virus. A mutation. I'm not really listening, but I hear the reporter's voice all the same. Viruses mutate all the time. Apparently, this means it's spreading more rapidly than before. The UK is being called Plague Island. I'm frightened for our families. I'm so frightened, all I can concentrate on are these drawings of bird shapes. Ghost shapes. Bird shapes. So many people are dying. So many are going to die. People we know, people we love. We are not able to travel, to be with them.

Don't cry.

Draw tick and v and m shapes. Large, medium, small. Swarm or flock. Flock of birds. Flock of ghosts. So many ghosts. Too many ghosts.

I draw a line of disappearing birds, making them smaller and smaller as they fly towards the left-hand corner of the paper.

Over the edge.

Away.

'Mrouwow. Mrououw.'

'Oh, Boy.' I unbolt the door again and let him in.

'Mrouow.'

'Stay in, this time.'

Bumping his head on the cat flap, he goes outside again.

The next time he comes in I crouch and stroke him. He purrs for a while. As I return to my drawing, spreading more wings, multiplying birds, he darts to the cat flap as if remembering something. He goes outside again.

Another lockdown. Now most of Europe is closing its borders to people from the UK. An irony, as the Brexit vote seemed to be mainly about keeping all the useful foreigners out.

I ask Morgan, 'Do you think one day we might have to decide to either stay here or go back—'

'It's not worth the risk.' Her gaze is fixed on the TV, she's focussed on the news.

'I guess now's not the time to make decisions.'

I wish there was just one family member here in New Zealand, for either of us.

From outside, 'Miouwurow.'

'Come on, then.' I open the door.

Boy comes in through the door and goes out through the cat flap again.

This goes on for some time.

Ink birds swarm across my page, splitting off, multiplying, flying solo, returning in wavering lines to dark-pencil clouds. From a distance, this drawing, all these swarming bird drawings I've been doing at night time recently, will look like magnified slides. Part of a brain, a neuron firing or misfiring. The edges of a plant cell, or the heart of it. No nucleus, all gales or water. Closer up, the drawings are unpredictable lines and clusters of hundreds of swarming, flocking, looping, ink birds.

'Miwrouw.'

Eventually Boy gives up on whatever it is he wants from me and drifts away into the night.

At this kitchen table if I draw all the birds
my dad ever saw when he was alive,
will the ghosts of those birds bring him to me?

As I fall asleep, I hover over my mum's house in Scotland. All the lights are off. It is not yet dawn.

My dad's fleece gardening jacket and cloth hat are still hanging on the back of his study door.

In his dark room, I lean my forehead against his hat.

I am divided.

Part of me is here in my dad's study leaning my head where his head once was.

Part of me is at the other end of the house, outside my mum's closed bedroom door. My hands are feathers as they gently stroke her fear from the air. I'm sending her a dream in which a flock of pencil-drawn birds catch the spreading virus in a net and carry it away from her.

'I miss you,' I whisper, to her closed bedroom door. 'So much. I'd do anything just to hug you.'

'I miss you,' I whisper, to the air inside his empty hat. 'Please come and find me. I'm still sure ghosts can travel as freely as they want to.'

In the morning, I open the glass doors. Outside on the deck beside the cat flap is a dead sparrow with no head. A gift from Boy.

Fingertipping my own neck, I examine the small blood-soaked

hole in the neck of this immigrant bird. Its tail feathers are dull and torn.

The feet are clenched as if its claws grip solid air.

Getting a tissue, I pick the headless bird up. I clasp it in my hands and carry it down the back steps into the garden.

A small burial, under the native kawakawa bush. I don't know the right or wrong words to say for the sparrow. What might this bird have believed in, if it believed in anything at all?

I try to cover all afterlife possibilities as I say, 'Travel well, be welcome in this earth, sleep sound, go to where you belong, fly to sparrow heaven, be whole again as a ghost bird, bless you, be with the loved ones you most miss, dream deep.'

And inside my throat I swallow the words, *don't be the bird my dad's ghost was travelling inside to find me. I'd recognise him, but only if I could see your face.*

After the bird's ineffective burial, everything is odd today. I am mouth-muffled and untalking. When I go to the supermarket to get milk, onions, coffee, strangers seem aggressive. They aren't really, but they're too physically close, too breathy, too loud. There's not enough air in this supermarket to hide the human-smells—perfume, smoke, sweat, garlic, shampoo. I am aware of hands touching trolleys, picking up cans, gripping baskets. Low voices are yellow sounds. More than anything I am aware of teeth, saliva, breath, movements of air. There's a distant cough from the next aisle and I try to remember what I came in to buy. Get in, get out. Another cough. Metal sound. Try not to make eye contact in case people speak and move even more air around.

It's safe here. So why feel like this?

This might be one of the few countries in the world with shops open this December. All shiny brightness. Tinsel. Glitter. Ribbon-wrapped high-heeled shoes and ribbon-wrapped boxes of chocolates. Perfume and whisky and aftershave and gin, bottles gleaming under shop-lights. With a flick of a plastic card against a machine we don't have to touch, we can pick up a piece of shiny brightness and take it home. Music spills from shop doorways. Familiar songs about snow and holly and winter blare out on this rainy summer's day. Most of the people are outside on the wet pavements, not inside the shops. Red and green figures flash to tell me when it's safe to cross the road. On outdoor café tables, forks shriek against plates. Laughter. And nearby, a cough. Can anything feel safe while our families in the UK are in so much danger?

Morgan's new studio is an industrial space divided by yellow lines on the floor. None of the other artists are in today. Morgan says the strip of rented space is *our* studio, not just hers. I've never had one before, so I don't know what to do yet. My bird drawings are at home on the kitchen table so I get my laptop out to write and sit on a yellow chair in the corner. There are overhead strip lights and the floor is painted bright-white. There are scratches and scuff marks everywhere. Morgan knows what to do, to make this a workable space. She clears unwanted papers into cardboard boxes, but we don't yet know where the recycling goes. She stacks the boxes in the centre of the space. She moves the desk to the window so light falls where she can use it.

The studio is on the fifth floor and the floors above and below are humming. An electric sound. A light blue-grey-green sound. Where does synaesthesia come from? The head or the body? I think about phantom limbs. What happens in the body, when the head is removed? Are the sensations of the head still felt, does the air it occupied still think for a while? Is there such a thing as a phantom-head?

Poor Boy. I buried his gift. A gift so delicious, he had to rip its head off. There is violence in some kinds of love. I try not to remember other times, other places, but feel more mouth-muffled than ever. I read about endangered stitchbirds and wish they really did stitch things together. I imagine them building nests, cottages, villages, castles, for future generations of themselves. I'm grateful for this ability we have, Morgan and I, to be silent together for hours, with neither of us minding or intruding. She's frowning at some old photos she's found in a box.

'Look,' she says. She shows me a handwritten poem. 'My mum wrote this when my dad died.'

It reveals the hopelessness of early grief. Scorings-out. Grief defining itself.

Morgan looks around, as if for something with an answer.

I say, 'I don't know what you should do with it either. Maybe just keep it safe.'

121

She places the poem in a desk drawer and slides it shut. Opening another box, she leans in and pulls out a pile of art books. She takes them out and puts them on a shelf.

The sound of sanding from the floor above. A deep rip—metal against wood. Stone judders against bone. I feel it in my jaw. I miss my mum and brothers. I feel the expansive curve of sky; from these grey sunlit clouds to their moon. How solid a jaw bone is. Vibrating with silence. Healthy. Strong. Guilty for being so safe. Frightened for those who aren't.

Two angled windows are ajar and a couple of inches of air comes in. There's a white sound—car wheels in the rain.

Between glass office blocks, there's a strip of blue-grey sea and a jetty containing multi-coloured shipping containers. I often wonder what's hidden inside them and about where they're destined to travel. We're only an hour's walk from home, but I'm missing our garden. How has it become possible to feel homesick for somewhere that's within walking distance? I'm missing the wide tree overcrowded with birds, only two fences away. There are nests in its leafiest branches. I saw a kingfisher in it once. All through the night, the branches are filled with roosting birds. At dawn and dusk the whole tree sings. There are so many bird-languages.

The overcrowded tree is a cathedral for birds.

Morgan says it's more like a block of flats.

Someone's voice in the corridor sounds light blue, interrupting silence, disappearing. A distant sneeze. Flash of amber.

'How do you want to get home?'

'On foot. The buses will be crowded.'

There are thousands of blocks of flats on Plague Island. So many people, living aggressively close. Side-by-side, up-and-down. No one can get in or out. And with more lockdowns coming, they're all of them in there, all of the time.

The block-of-flat-cathedral-tree full of birds won't miss one headless sparrow.

Someone should be missing it.

When we're back at home, there's post. Morgan flicks the kettle on and opens an envelope which contains an academic journal. While she sits down to read, I go outside into the garden.

Kneeling at the base of the kawakawa bush, I whisper, 'I am so sorry for not understanding what the yowls of a cat meant. But if the headless sparrow was you, it was probably already too late. Is occupying a bird called possessing or haunting or reincarnation or recycling? Were you inside the head or the heart, or only the wings? Did you fly away in the poor sparrow's moment of death? If that was your next life or your first attempt at bird-possession, I'm sorry it ended before I got to see your face.

Please, fly here to me again—there are so many pairs of wings for you to choose from. You can move around here more freely than people can in the UK, though we all have survivor-guilt. I guess whatever country we're in, lockdown is irrelevant for ghosts.

Till you come back I'll draw pictures for you; flocks of birds which are also flocks of ghosts. My hands make beckoning movements, while drawing. I'll keep drawing and drawing and drawing in case ghosts understand the murmuring languages of pencil, lead, and ink.'

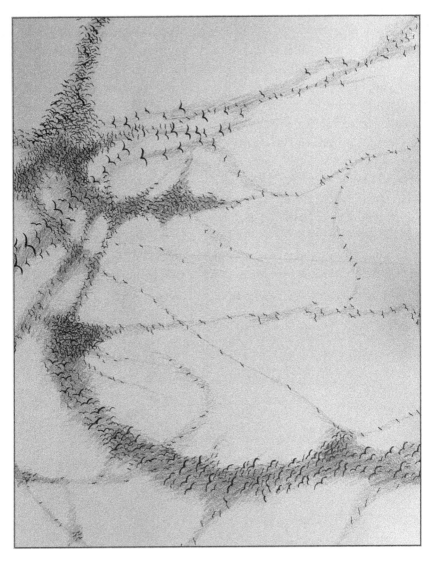

Flock of Ghosts I

Airborne, Spreading, Silent

During the first lockdown I have guilt for feeling anything that isn't about loss or fear, death and grieving. Surely these are the only appropriate emotions for this strange time. But there's also an overwhelming sense of relief because I'm no longer trying to force myself to connect with the other people who live in this city.

Now, to protect each other and ourselves, we have to stay at home. In the silent air between me and Morgan I can rest like a shadow, like snow, like some tired echo. And what will happen, when there is silence?

I'll have space to wonder why it is so hard for me to connect with people, even though I'm highly empathic. I'll realise I've felt lonely my whole life, even when I was surrounded by familiar people.

I don't know why.

Now no one is annoyed with me when I say, 'I don't know' I can let myself think about what it is I don't know. Like a whispered idea that there's something there, something I should try harder to understand.

I whisper, 'But what is it?'

No reply. Not yet.

Eight Words for Loneliness

Despane– The loneliness of feeling misunderstood, unloved or unheard by someone who used to understand, love or listen.

Starn– Craving something or someone to be there but knowing it's/ they're not. Wanting to bite something.

Youache– Where a specific person is missed and only their physical presence will cure the ache of missing them.

Ignornly– The kind of loneliness that other people notice, but don't mention to the person they think is lonely. Their expression shows sympathy, but also a little wariness, as if loneliness could be contagious.

Solilone– A type of melancholia experienced while gazing at a wide-skied landscape. A longing for strangeness, for the unreal or the surreal to appear.

Idealone– A hankering for an imagined scenario—where it's the idea of the situation that causes the loneliness. For example, the 'ideal' of the perfect friend sitting opposite on the sofa, laughing over wine and confessions and saying all of the right things.

Achiposs– The ache of missing out on experiencing something beautiful, because it is impossible.

Disampty– Where the immediate environment is problematic – usually in practical ways. The rubbish split all over the floor, the smoke alarm is going off, work is waiting, the clock is ticking, the umbrella's broken, it's lashing with rain and there's no one else around.

The Ghost Sanctuary

My dad worked too hard, for too long, with too many difficulties. I wish he'd retired much earlier but none of us knew he'd die suddenly at the age of sixty-seven. Sometimes I am transported back into his past, into difficult memories.

I want to stay here in the present because I am lucky—Morgan and I have made a loving home together in New Zealand. We are both artists and writers. She's been a successful academic for many years and recently did a PhD just because she wanted one. I teach creative writing in classrooms or online and am lucky that I can earn money by giving people advice about the stories they want to write.

Tonight as we eat the mushroom soup I've made for dinner, Morgan tells me about her other memories of work—of the time she spent working on archaeological digs back in the UK. The digging and recording techniques were different to the Egyptian methods we've just seen on the telly. As far as we could tell, the Egyptian archaeologists didn't record the layers of soil or rock, or use grids, but instead, dug down, pulled out sand-covered artefacts and cleaned them with delicate brushes. Morgan suspects it's because the soil in the UK is wet and claggy compared to desert sand.

I look at the kitchen floorboards, imagining them one day being gradually revealed by delicate brushes from beneath layers of soil or sand. Not long after we first moved in, Morgan filled the holes in these floorboards and then painted the floorboards wood-colours again. She used the lines and tones of real wood. If there are archaeologists in the future, this floor will be really confusing for them.

Are memories buried in different textures within our minds? Claggy for the dark and sticky memories we don't want to think about. Fine sand for memories we want to dust off and examine. Perhaps it's *because* I feel contented with Morgan, it feels safe to time-travel back to the claggier memories of my dad.

What if in the process of remembering, these memories can be transformed—for his sake and my own?

Memory:

My dad has four children and a wife and goats and cats and chickens and ducks and a house to keep, all on a primary-school teacher's salary. Damp patches mottle the hallway walls and the roof leaks onto the bathroom floor. There are buckets in the attic and when we swing on the wonky banister, we can hear drips. Slates can be fixed, but the winds are fierce here and a strong gust will find any loose ones the costly roofer hasn't. Next year, when the bank loan is cleared and a new one can be applied for, a damp course will be done. Many years later, the roof will be replaced.

Transformation:

I am the wind, calming a gale by blowing through it. The gale is pushed in another direction, so instead of breaking more slates, it blows moss off the gutters. My dad picks up a moss-clump and examines it as if it were a miniature velvet island. As he leaves for work at eight in the morning he puts it in his jacket pocket. He thumbs it gently throughout his day.

Memory:

We live in the country and my dad teaches six miles away at Kirkcolm Primary School. He has a boom-voice loud enough to summon a whole school of playful kids in from the playground. In his classroom, he teaches seven to nine-year-olds maths and recorder music. He teaches reading and singing. He teaches art and spelling and sciences and weather. How it rains, and why. My brothers and I all pass through his class. I overlap with my older brother who's a genius at maths but for me numbers jumble up and make no sense. Maths makes clouds come into the classroom and get sucked into my head when we're meant to do sums. When it's not maths I pay more attention. My dad punishes me sometimes. All the teachers have to, because I can't get maths right. But at night when I'm crying over homework, he shows me how to hide my mistakes by drawing over the wrong numbers with daisy-like flowers. I keep doing this and often my homework is a whole page of mistake-flowers.

Transformation:

While my dad struggles to teach me maths. I look up from my desk and tell him, 'There's nothing wrong with the way you're teaching, it's just I have maths-clouds in my head.' I say, 'But it's not your fault. When I grow up, I'll be good at writing and drawing because I don't mind making mistakes. Mistake-flowers can grow into all kinds of unexpected things, when I water them enough.' He smiles, but I can tell he either didn't hear me, or doesn't believe what I said, yet.

Memory:

My dad takes his pupils for walks in nature—along the path beside the school that leads into the woods. When outside the school grounds my dad teaches us with an attitude of serious playfulness, a determined expression on an unsmiling face as he points at a green bank, showing us something he wants us to understand. He frowns, waiting for a particular reaction. When he sees surprise or delight in our faces as we understand how ferns unfurl much like lizards or kittens or snakes might, his face softens into a wide-lipped smile. He teaches us how to identify different types of trees from the shapes of their leaves. Oak, willow, beech. Back in the classroom he teaches us what birds-of-prey can and can't digest by examining the droppings of owls. We examine the punctured corpses of voles while he teaches us how birds-of-prey kill.

At home my dad shuts himself in his study and prepares lessons and marks homework late into the nights. All around him, piled high, are papers and books, stationery and cardboard boxes, craft materials and files. He rises early and checks through everything he's done the night before. One year he discovers from talking to the children in his class that most of them don't have advent calendars. He wants to take the battered calendars we four children have collected over the years and give them to all the children in his class. 'You have far too many,' he says. 'You don't need them all.' I think some of the children at school might be lying. He reluctantly lets us claw back one or two favourites, but now I feel guilty whenever I open an advent calendar door. I don't know who was lying and who was telling the truth. A quiet truthful kid who didn't shout over a loud lying one might have loved this picture of a red-wrapped gift under door number 3. Or under double-door number 24, another truthful kid would have loved the magical glow in the air over the baby's crib.

Transformation:

As an adult, I stand invisibly next to my dad in his classroom. I whisper in his ear not to trust that everyone tells the truth. I whisper, 'You need to look at their eyes, to know for certain.' His head tilts, listening, but he can't hear my voice. I put my hand gently on his back and stand silently beside him all day.

Memory:

My dad keeps himself hidden away at weekends, marking and marking and marking. I come to realise over time that his job must remind him of his angry father's sharp eyes and blunt hands, waiting for the moment to strike. My dad can't drop his guard. He can't let himself make mistakes. At Kirkcolm Primary School there are a few angry fathers who think my dad isn't tough enough on their kids because he won't use the belt. They also dislike him because he's an Englishman living in Scotland and a vegetarian among beef farmers. He's not to be trusted because he has long hair and a beard, he wears odd waistcoats and patchwork trousers, he has a wife who's not interested in Tupperware or the Women's Institute and four is far too many children for someone who won't say if they're a Catholic or not.

Over time, my dad gets all four belts removed from all four classrooms of Kirkcolm Primary School. The angry fathers find something else to complain about. They now they want their children to be taught to fear a protestant god rather than being taught to fear badly played recorder music, landslides or particular types of poisonous mushrooms.

I'm told by a kid on the school bus that my dad seems Good but he must really be Bad because he believes Rocks have Souls. I shrug it off and ask my dad about this later on. He laughs and says, 'Well, rocks *might* have souls.'

'How?' I reply.

'How, or why?' With a glint in his eyes, he asks this confusing question. In the local dialect that used to be called Gallow-Irish before the troubles started, *how* means *why*. I don't know if my dad also knows this, or if it's just me and my brothers who understand the dialect we've had to learn. We speak Gallow-Irish at school and English at home. My parents' voices are always the same no matter who they're speaking to. My dad saying *how or why* confuses me so much I don't remember the conversation about the souls of rocks ever being resolved.

Transformation:

I hand my dad a rock. The rock falls through his ghost hand and lands on the floorboards with a bang.

His ghost looks at the rock with a slightly surprised expression.

I ask him in my loudest voice, 'Does a Rock have a Soul?'

This time he hears me. He laughs and says, 'Of course not. A rock has solidity. But don't underestimate the value of solidity.' He examines the transparency of his hands. 'You don't need to understand maths, to understand that.'

Memory:
Our black and white telly gets BBC Northern Ireland because it's the nearest signal, though we're in Scotland. Across the Irish Sea, bombs go off. We hear them and don't hear them. The Right Reverend Ian Paisley rants on our television and my mum does impressions of his raging voice. Margaret Thatcher stops milk deliveries to primary schools and she is also on the telly but never at exactly the same time as The Right Reverend Ian Paisley. I often wonder if they are secretly the same person.

The goats try to eat our t-shirts and towels off the washing line. We tether them to poles. Our horned goat Ruby butts my youngest brother too near his eye. There's a lot of shrieking and a lot of blood. Ruby's amber eyes can't tell the difference between small humans and tall humans. Either that or she can, which means she's pure evil. After the attack my parents take her away to live with someone else. We don't see her again.

At secondary school a mean-eyed boy tells me he's got Ruby at his farm and he kicks her all the time.

I twist his short hair between my knuckles and he retaliates by pulling me outside by my wrist. I end up on top of him on the concrete surface of the playground, fist raised. A teacher drags me off him. When I'm on my feet, the teacher yells down at him, 'Boys don't fight with girls!'

I'm almost sorry for the boy because he's smaller than me.

He doesn't mention Ruby again.

Transformation:
My little brother's face doesn't carry a scar. Ruby the goat has grown white wings and a halo. At Christmas my dad dresses her up in a chewed blue t-shirt and wraps white towels around her horns. Beneath door 24 of the advent calendar, Ruby's got the glowing-holy-virgin role in the primary school nativity play. She drinks

ghost-milk from bottles gifted by a ghost called The Wrong Margaret Reverend Thatcher. The milk is a thank-you gift to my dad for getting rid of the four belts at school.

Memory:
My dad often meets ex-pupils who are all grown up in the local town. Many of them introduce him to their children and tell him how much he meant to them. But on the few occasions when a complaint is made against him, his voice changes and he sounds like a small boy.

His voice doesn't falter when threats are made outside his work. One night a man tries to axe his way through our gate. Me and my middle brother watch him from our bedroom window which overlooks the front of the house. After falling over, the man retrieves his axe and staggers away, cursing. When we tell our parents about it, our dad says they watched the man from the kitchen window. We ask why they didn't chase him away or call the police. He explains, 'We're not worried about anyone who's too drunk to open an unlocked gate.'

Transformation:
I summon the axe man's ghost mother. She arrives with a scratchy blanket and wraps the axe man up. She takes the axe man home and gives him black coffee to sip on. While she looks after him, I become a ghost too as I swaddle his axe in bedsheets and tell him to go to sleep.

Memory:
When I am a teenager on a night out in the local town, my dad rescues me and a male friend from an aggressive man. My dad gets out of his car, opens the back door and shouts at us to get in. The aggressive man releases his grip on my friend's neck, takes his eyes off my face, turns and locks eyes with my dad. My friend and I rush away into the car. My dad doesn't break eye-contact with the man while he too gets into the car and drives

off. Years later, the same man ends up doing time in prison for murder. I still feel guilty, wondering what would have happened if he'd attacked my dad. The man's nickname was Flea and I never knew his real name. Flea physically attacked every male he saw me speaking to, or got his gang to attack them on his behalf. He never once touched me.

Transformation:

I write Flea a ghost-love-letter in invisible ink, but don't sign it, because all these love-words are lies.

I place it under the flat pillow in his cell and hope the blank page brings him some comfort on the nights he can't sleep.

Memory:

Long after I've left home, my dad takes early retirement in the final year it's offered. He gets another job teaching childcare courses at the local tech college. Some of the students have been sent there as an alternative to going on the dole and have no interest in caring for anyone at all, let alone children. A couple of teenagers are bored. In long corridors they talk about falsely accusing either a tutor or the janitor of hitting one of them. Accusing a tutor will gain them more attention than accusing the janitor, so they accuse my dad. When the other students eventually realise my dad is suspended and why, they speak up about these overheard conversations and my dad's name is cleared. But when I phone him, his voice is strained and remains so. He doesn't understand lying, though I try to explain it to him.

His tears rarely, if ever, fall. They build up inside him like an ocean with no safe place to go to. His voice that could boom at a school-full of noisy kids is squashed into the voice of a small boy. Even as his voice gradually strengthens, he sounds tired each time I phone him. There's something about lying which damages how he sees people, the world. Himself perhaps. Because he seems so small, in our conversations I mention vast and bright things that won't ever harm him. Stars, the moon's phases, the sunrise and sunset. But right now he can't imagine the brightness of anything. Whatever dark feelings he has about lies, I can't get him to speak with me about them.

Transformation:

I meet my dad's ghost in a forest. We sit together on a fallen tree. I hold out a transparent bowl and catch all my dad's unshed tears. Once he's cried them all out, I cover the bowl with a lid made from woven twigs and leave him in the forest for a while. I climb a cliff and throw the bowl into a dark ocean.

When I arrive back in the forest, he's walking along a muddy path, smiling at the absence of his own footprints. He tells me my skin is as pale as a ghost and asks me where the bowl of his tears has gone. I tell him his tears had ambitions to travel instead of staying still, 'So they've gone off to sail the seas in a lying boat.'

'What's a lying boat?' He stops walking to look at a lichen-covered rock.

I reply, 'A sanctuary for birds to sleep on half-way across an ocean, when they're tired from their migrations. It gives them somewhere to rest—which stops so many of them dying on the way.'

I glance at him and smile. 'Sometimes people lie because they need a break from relentlessly telling the truth. Or so they can better understand the limits of their choices. Or so they can feel important instead of insignificant. But... back to the birds, the boat and the tears which are now travelling away from you. Only birds can see the lying boat, because it's made of thin layers of keratin, the substance forming their beaks, feathers and claws. You taught me about keratin, at primary school.'

I can hear the smile in his voice as he says, 'You remember.'

Memory:

My mum does the household sums and tells my dad that now is a safe time to finally retire. She shows him the same sums again and again, understanding he needs time. Understanding he needs to be certain everything will be all right.

Even after he's retired, he still keeps the things he'd collected for work. His study and all the cupboards and attics and sheds are filled with paints and brushes, musical instruments, multi-coloured paper, lesson plans, child development theory books and stress management texts. One cupboard contains his collection of bones. Another, percussion instruments. My mum tries and fails to get him to clear the over-stuffed shelves again, again, again. When I visit, at her request I go into his study with a black binbag, 'To help him.' He goes so pale and quiet at the thought at throwing anything out, I can't bear to force him. We move things instead, shifting books from one cupboard into another. Eventually he volunteers a few cardboard files, 'To be destroyed—they've got names on them.'

Transformation:

I'm standing outside their house in the dark. There's a new moon and it's the hour before dawn. I'm a ghost-witch, singing a wild song towards the horizon. The wind rises and with it comes the sea. A great wave washes through my parent's house while they're still asleep. Their double bed floats and falls as the wave recedes. They wake in a far emptier home. The objects left behind are the ones which are most significant. My dad's camera and photographs. The bottle of morning dew he gave my mum on her birthday. The patchwork wall-hanging she made from our old clothes. My mum is content and without sentiment. My dad has sentiment, but is willing to forget. He glances at me and says, 'This kind of travel is dangerous, you know. Neither here, nor there. You're so pale you're almost invisible. Better not stay much longer.'

Memory:
My dad volunteers at the local bird sanctuary, one day a week. It's not just birds he's keeping an eye on though. When I spend the day with him there, he sits at a trestle table with a collection of small tubs with holes in the lids. Rain clatters on the shed roof. He's counting live moths. These were caught the night before by using light boxes. Once he's identified and counted all the different types of moths, they'll be released. While he's busy, I walk along the cliffs. Herring gulls wheel over white-crested waves and rain batters the walls of a whitewashed lighthouse. This is a true sanctuary—an isolated peninsula, all sky, cliffs and ocean. I imagine the moths in those tubs my dad is holding. Breathing through airholes. Longing for flight.

Transformation:
The bird sanctuary has become not only a sanctuary for birds and moths, but for all kinds of ghosts. At the Ghost Sanctuary, no one is paid a salary, so no one has authority over my dad's ghost. He's free to come and go as he pleases. I've become a ghost moth and am inside one of those tubs his ghost is holding. When he opens my tub, I flutter out and land on his fingernail. He leans forwards and examines me closely, considering what kind of moth I might be. I flex my wings and hope his ghost will be curious enough to grow some wings of his own. The eerie sound of a herring gull calls us outside. As he opens the door, I hover over his hand and when we're out on the cliffs, I land on his outstretched fingertip.

At the bottom of the cliffs, waves wash one way and slosh back.

Ghost cormorants stand on the rocks, drying their wing-cloaks in the wind.

In the sky, clouds veil a full moon and the wild Irish sea is hidden in shadows.

My dad holds me close to his green eye and says, 'I'm

quite safe here, but it's not home for you. Go,' he murmurs. 'Before you vanish.'

Moths need a single light source. Our miniature wings desire brightness. That's what instinct really is—a small part of us recognises the right direction and rushes towards it.

Love pulls at me from beyond this dark horizon. Clouds slide away and reveal a bright moon.

All around the Ghost Sanctuary, wings whirr.

Morgan's voice, 'Be here now, with me.' As I return, she's beside me on the sofa, reading a novella with the word Feathers in the title[3].

Tonight there's a large moth fluttering and whirring around. Morgan is afraid of moths. I usually catch them and put them outside. Despite walking around the kitchen extending my cupped hands, this one is impossible to catch.

It appears and disappears.

In the morning, it's lying dead on the painted floorboards.

Its delicate wings are as pale as my skin.

2020
Cancelled Flight

How far from their graves, can ghosts travel?
Grave-width? Soil-depth? Cloud-height?
How far from their nests, can birds travel?
Ocean-width? Grass-depth? Sun-height?
The borders are still closed.
Flights are cancelled.
The sky is cancelled.
Flowers on his grave are cancelled.
Hugging my mum is cancelled.
Talking into the air over his bones is cancelled.
Only in dreams, is it still possible to fly.

---

3   Max Porter, *Grief is the Thing with Feathers.*

Three Friends

F and I met because he came to my creative writing classes for local adults in Wellington. At the end of his eight-week course, he emailed me to tell me why he showed up in the first place. Something to do with reading one of my novels because his mum didn't want to. This made me laugh. He also emailed me to tell me he appreciated me for treating everyone in the classroom exactly the same. We meet around once every six months. We send each other messages on our phones to check in on writing and life things. The friendship takes place almost entirely on the Messenger app. In this way, I talk to F more frequently than anyone else I've met here. The few times we've met up in person he didn't make much eye contact, but tried to. F is a brilliant writer who loves cats and dishwashers and knows a lot about different kinds of pegs.

When I first came to New Zealand a UK writer sent me E's email as someone I might like to make friends with. E had just left Australia to move back to New Zealand because she'd become too sick to work. Kiwis can't sign on in Australia, though Australians can sign on in New Zealand. I like E because she's kind and funny and gentle, she's a good writer, and she really loves Morgan. Though that's not a remarkable thing—everyone I've introduced to Morgan really loves her. E comes to our house about three or four times a year, usually around birthday-times. I've seen photos of her home. She has gorilla bookends and a dinosaur lamp.

D is an artist who lives a few miles outside Wellington. We met because Morgan taught her when she was doing her masters degree and D has read and liked all three of my books. I love her paintings. The ones I've seen in real life rather than as photographs were in a gallery, long before the pandemic. They were colourful paintings of dark and twisted characters from fairy tales. There was one with a crow, a human heart and a cage. Looking at it, my guts clenched and my shoulder blades had the sensation of wings, unfurling. I meet D about once every six months for a coffee and we talk about her life and my life and her paintings and my writing. We laugh a lot.

Though I don't usually eat cake, I almost always eat cake when I'm with D. So whenever I think of her, I think of paint and flour and murky water and ginger and fairy tales and brown sugar and the textures of paintbrush bristles.

Now Covid is spreading in New Zealand, everyone's hiding. I don't know when I'll see any of these three people who were slowly becoming close friends. Or G, who I was also wanting to make friends with too. I really like G because she's an interesting and brave writer and she's always kind to the students. I still work with her sometimes, but only online.

Time has gone strange again. Last week feels like last month. Six months ago must be at least a year ago. My dad was only sixty-seven when he died. Covid has been spreading for months or years or days. Decades? My dad died Before-Covid. So many people are dying Of-Covid or With-Covid or During-Covid. In London there is a grey wall filled with thousands of red love hearts with their names on them. It is not yet After-Covid. Perhaps it the virus will be with us forever now, as Always-Covid. Somewhere in the future, it's 2060AC. Everyone who's left, wherever they live in the world, always has Covid.

I don't know when I last saw anyone I'm related to. Dates and years are all jumbled up.

People all around us are only seeing their families, necessary work colleagues, or the closest of friends.

It's so easy to slip away into shadows.

I was almost becoming visible while I was still trying to make friends here.

Morgan's friends check in on her, mainly via text messaging as she doesn't want to risk getting Covid.

I have to keep her safe, which means I can't see anyone either.

From what I've read from many wise women who know these things, women disappear as we get older[4]. And right now everyone is getting older, too fast.

When Morgan's not around I often feel like a ghost.

---

4 "…now others look straight through you, you are completely invisible to them, you have become a ghost." Mary Ruefle, *Pause*.

I wonder how many people all over the world are living like this.

Conspiracy theorists shout loudest, but this shouting seems to happen almost entirely online. So they're probably indoors writing social media posts about having the freedom to go outside. With a bit of practice, social media is easily ignored.

Ghosting.

Don't breathe. Don't touch. Don't notice the lack of breath or touch.

Are we only real when someone looks at us?

To Butterfly a Ghost

Preheat the sunshine to 67 degrees centigrade.

Feel the air around you to locate a ghost and make sure it is either asleep or sedated.

If the ghost already has wings, release it immediately.

Assuming there are no wings; using sharp kitchen shears, remove the spine from the ghost.

Dust the spine with flour and cut it into small pieces. Set the spine aside.

Flatten the ghost by placing it face-up on the floor and applying firm pressure to the chest air.

Transfer the flattened ghost to a wire-rack.

Drizzle the ghost with olive oil.

Combine salt, black pepper and baking powder in a small bowl. Sprinkle this mixture over the ghost.

Smother the ghost with herb leaves: sage, parsley, thyme.

Lie the ghost in sunshine to roast, until a thermometer inserted into the thickest part of the ghost registers 67 degrees centigrade.

Immediately reduce the heat of the sun if the ghost darkens.

Heat one tablespoon of oil in a small saucepan until the oil is shimmering.

Add the ghost spine and cook, stirring frequently for 67 minutes.

Add onion, carrot, celery, bay leaves, vermouth or sherry and one cup of water.

Stir this mixture with a wooden spoon. Reduce the heat and simmer for 67 minutes.

Blend the mixture and boil it for another 67 minutes. Whisk in soy sauce, butter and lemon juice to make a jus.

Remove the butterflied ghost from the sunshine, transfer it to the floor.

Feed it the spine jus. Tell it that once it has mastered independent flight, it will learn speech.

Wrap the ghost loosely in foil and let it rest.

Release it outside and watch it fly away north.

Make a final attempt at a beckoning wish. Think of the white-skied north. Whisper, 'Come hither.' Ask the ghost to return soon with the ghost of your father: because it chooses to, because it has empathy for you, because it must. Because you have used a cooking spell to give it wings.

Keep your eyes on the sky.

Lose your appetite when the butterflied ghost never comes back.

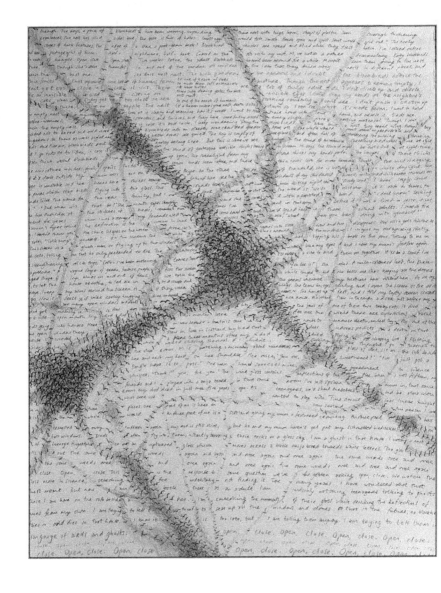

Flock of Ghosts II

Nine Words for Loneliness

Despane– The loneliness of feeling misunderstood, unloved or unheard by someone who used to understand, love or listen.

Starn– Craving something or someone to be there but knowing it's/they're not. Wanting to bite something.

Youache– Where a specific person is missed and only their physical presence will cure the ache of missing them.

Ignornly– The kind of loneliness that other people notice, but don't mention to the person they think is lonely. Their expression shows sympathy, but also a little wariness, as if loneliness could be contagious.

Solilone– A type of melancholia experienced while gazing at a wide-skied landscape. A longing for strangeness, for the unreal or the surreal to appear.

Idealone– A hankering for an imagined scenario—where it's the idea of the situation that causes the loneliness. For example, the 'ideal' of the perfect friend sitting opposite on the sofa, laughing over wine and confessions and saying all of the right things.

Achiposs– The ache of missing out on experiencing something beautiful, because it is impossible.

Disampty– Where the immediate environment is problematic – usually in practical ways. The rubbish split all over the floor, the smoke alarm is going off, work is waiting, the clock is ticking, the umbrella's broken, it's lashing with rain and there's no one else around.

Crowdsad– Felt while around many other people. Crying while walking along streets crammed with strangers, feeling unable to speak during a burbling conversation in which others are talking loudly and not leaving any gaps.

Empathy Splinters

I'm not ready for this.

Today, I'm going outside and I'll be around strangers. I should have practised in advance, but I didn't. I'm going to read at a literary festival event in the city centre. I've done reading events before, but not for a while. Being around a lot of new people all at the same time is like being static while colours and smells and thoughts and pictures and sounds I've not chosen move chaotically around me.

It's hard to work out what belongs where.

As I walk to the event, I try to plant my feet firmly on the pavements of Adelaide Road, then all around the Basin Reserve and onto Cuba. I have to remind myself what my role is, because this will also help me to blank out the chaos. I am a writer, a listener, a smiler. I will be within a group of writers I haven't met, in an alleyway outside a bookshop. We'll be reading to an audience of people who like books.

The paving stones spot with rain as people walk past me. Their voices trail through the air behind them as lines of colours. Pink. Green. Brown.

I'm not ready for this.

But it will be all right. I can leave as soon as it's over. Many reading events like this take place all over this city. There won't be too many people there because of social distancing rules. Each event lasts forty-five minutes. No one is entirely sure yet how the virus is transmitted. We're wearing masks everywhere because if it travels via breath, it's airborne. We should be safe outside, or wherever air isn't trapped.

There are crowds on Cuba Street. Masks cover faces from the eyes down. I pause in a doorway and change my black fabric mask to a thin surgical mask. The information sheet from the events team said they were easier for reading.

The smell of ginger. White. The smell of men's deodorant. Grey. The smell of hand cream. Turquoise.

Everything's a bit too vivid.

I've been indoors for too long. I should have practiced going outside before now. I should also have practiced reading through a mask. I turn into the mall and head towards the second-hand bookshop we're reading outside. Morgan will be reading at a different event later on this evening. Hers will be a few streets away from here, inside a dusty office building. I wonder if these surgical masks protect us from dust as well as germs. What about sand, gas, bad smells, pollen, spores? All the airborne things. My mouth is covered by a paper-thin hand.

Masks are a way of keeping people safe, especially when there are no vaccines. But it's so hard to feel safe around people in masks. I don't want to look into their eyes, but I have to. Otherwise how will I know who's dangerous? I'm searching people's eyes or bodies for what I would usually see in their faces.

It's Saturday evening at twenty to six which is exactly the time I've been asked to arrive. I'm greeted by a masked woman with a clipboard and I tick a form to tell her that *yes, I am very well, quite well, completely well, happy to comply, all my own responsibility, masks and hand sanitiser, yes and thank you.*

She ushers me past trestle tables stacked with boxes of books. Under some birdshit-stained awnings are a row of mismatched chairs and a waiting microphone. I sit in the middle and look up at the beams, seeking the birds I can hear but not see. I practice wearing my reading glasses with my mask and even outside in the cold, they steam up. I keep trying but they mist and don't clear. I wipe them again. They mist and don't clear. I can't breathe and see at the same time. I try again. And again.

A small crowd of masked people arrive outside the bookshop in pairs, arranging themselves around the trestle tables. The audience doesn't have chairs. The ground is shiny and there's damp in the air. Everything is concrete-cold. I hope we start on time and finish early, so the audience can all sit down soon, somewhere else, somewhere with warm food and blankets.

Another writer in a surgical mask arrives and the air around her is all black and velvety, so I know she's soft enough to be safe. She's got slick dark hair and brown eyes and asks me if I'm reading one poem or two.

I muffle a reply through my mask, 'I'm reading prose. For about six mi—'

She turns away as another writer arrives. The second writer is the texture of pink threads. They hug each other with odd precision. Slotted in. Slotted out.

'Hey! Did you hear C couldn't come,' the velvety one says, 'Because she's having a baby?'

'Good excuse.'

I put my reading glasses in my coat pocket and think about how hopeful it is that parents are still having babies during a pandemic. The babies might not come out though, if they decide they'd be safer in the womb. The world is getting scary. I imagine pregnant bodies growing to the size of giants so they can contain their unbirthed offspring: babies to toddlers to children to teenagers to adults.

Our Host, Hope, arrives. It's not her real name but it suits her. She's got lush black hair and confident legs. Her eyes shine as I introduce myself. She shakes my hand and laughs about having emailed me a tarot card I didn't like, in advance of this event. We were all sent a card, to prompt the writing we'll read tonight.

I smile behind my mask but can't catch her eye because she's looking past me at the other writers, 'Did you hear about C?' she says to them.

They all talk about C and the advice she's had about when exactly her baby might be born. Not for another month, apparently, but she's got to be in bed all that time. The pink thread writer says, 'They've got to stay still.'

It must be strange to be two people, temporarily.

The air around me shifts and shifts back again. A prickle to the skin.

The final writer arrives and she is red and black. She approaches me. I introduce myself and ask where she's from. She hears my voice and calls me English and I tell her I'm more Scottish than English and she calls me English again. I stop talking.

She sits beside the black velvet writer.

The masked audience shift in front of us all. Negotiating gaps, advancing and retreating, moving their hips, shoulders, feet.

Where to stand. How? Here. Stand between me and her, if you can.
I don't want to feel this. Please don't feel this with me. Don't look at me.

Who thinks this? Me or them?

All the writers are seated and I'm still in the middle. I should have sat at the edge nearest the microphone, then I could have hidden behind whoever was talking.

What would happen to the two writers talking to each other on my right and the two talking to each other on my left if I suddenly vanished? Would the pairs topple into each other, falling into the space my body left behind?

I'm feeling too much that isn't mine. Jagged, a small split to the upper spine. A crack, opening.

If I become invisible, the other writers might think I am still here until they swivel their eyes in my direction. They can share the warmth of my body sitting here between them, sense the breath-moisture I'm wiping away yet again from my reading glasses.

A plump pigeon lands near my feet. I slip my glasses back in my pocket and whisper hello to it. Leaning forwards I smile, watching it waddle.

I'm completely invisible and imagine the four writers have just noticed. They're saying:

'How odd I thought there was someone—'
'No, there was. But—'
'There are meant to be five of us, aren't there?'
'Which one was she?'
'Do you know her—'
'I don't. Do you?'

The young woman with the clipboard comes up to us and says, 'OK, ready to go. Hope—you ready to test the mic and get chairing?'

I reappear.

The pigeon has disappeared in the shadows beneath a table. I want to crawl in after it.

Behind my mask I smile at Hope's white 1960s platform boots with red love hearts all over them.

She tells the audience that they'll hear some new writing about a tarot card which she drew for each of us in advance. She says my name.

Clasping my pages to read from, I get up and approach the

microphone. I'm relieved finally to be reading because this means the event will be over soon and I can go home.

I try to link my writing to the tarot card Hope drew for me; the Three of Swords. The card shows a picture of a heart with three swords plunged through it. A crowd of faces I can't see watch me. I tell them I'll read two short pieces of writing. Muffled, through a mask, through a microphone. One piece of my writing is sort-of about 'rules of three' but it's really about a homeless ghost and three fat pigeons. The other is about the human heart as a bird and as a musical instrument.

Loose connections.

I try to feel my own words as I read, squint-eyed. It seems pointless to read to people when I can't see their faces. I can't tell if they're interested or not. Should I cut it short? Only read one? I said I'd read two. So, I read two.

I'm a ghost, reading to ghosts.

The plump pigeon wanders past again and it's brought a friend. I don't want to look at masked faces any more, so I read my writing to the pigeons.

When I finish, the sound of clapping startles them back into the shadows.

Hope introduces the next two writers who read beautiful poems based on The World and the Page of Cups. I examine their feet as they read. Pretty witch shoes. Black strappy sandals. These are not the kinds of shoes you can run away in. They must have known they wouldn't want to.

When the red and black writer gets up to read, she tells the audience that she didn't allow Hope to choose a tarot card for her, but chose her own. She wears soft gypsy-style clothing, silks and cottons. Dressing gown over layers.

She tells us that she always draws The Tower whenever she casts her own tarot cards.

So she's chosen to write about this card.

The one card I hoped no one would be talking about.

The Tower. Solid walls, cracking. Crumbling to rubble. Complete destruction.

In the weeks leading up to the breakup with my ex-wife Z, I was casting my own tarot cards. The Tower appeared at the bottom, in position ten. Each time I cast my cards, it appeared higher up the spread. Getting nearer and nearer to the present moment. I knew The Tower was coming. I was fearful of what it meant. That's the nature of The Tower, its destructive inevitability.

On the day it arrived in the top position, the breakup happened. This is how I remember it:

Z's ultimatum. My answer. Shouting. My silence. A lot of shouting. Silence. More shouting. Then the longest silence.

Everything changed.

I rang my dad first. I didn't know what else to do, so I told him what had happened. It helped to make it real, to make it definite. In our family marriages last, no matter what private difficulties there are. I needed to hear that he and my mum still loved me.

Then I ran away. Kept running. Didn't stop till I got here, to Morgan.

Cracks and holes tremble invisibly in the air as the red and black woman speaks. I'm not sure if I'm really seeing her, or half-seeing Z. Her words are emotive, passionate, bored, honest. Brutally so. She talks of suicide. She is no longer the writer at this festival, she is memory. She is how I remember. She is The Tower. She is a mood shift, she is talk and distract. Look at me. Look over there. The Tower has collapsing edges—it seeps and leaks and spreads and collapses, leaving vertical absence, filling horizontal space with detritus. She is oil and water and splitting. I try to imagine her mask and my mask as shields but her eyes flash. Z's eyes flash with anger and distress. I don't know who I'm seeing, but terrible things have happened, at all ages and stages of her life. I try to look away so I can avoid seeing them. There's a bitter smell I don't recognise, hidden beneath floral perfume. I try to hear the writer, but it's hard to see past The Tower. Stone walls, cracking. Images inside sounds. There are strong shoulders. Lies. Threats, smoke, cracks in beams, in glass. Small rooms containing clutters of strange ornaments and bright-painted furniture and ex-lovers lying in crumpled bedlinen. Impossible ultimatums. Torn notebooks. Blocked. Ghosted. Ex-lovers as dried out empty shells.

Her eyes above her mask gleam with a smile, but shift into anger. Whose eyes am I seeing?

I'm not ready for this.

This is not how I want to remember.

I'm staring at the concrete floor again.

The audience is listening. For a moment I leave myself and thread myself through their shoulders like mist, to listen with them. She's talking about boredom and how dull most men and some women are.

A memory of being told about ex-lovers being destroyed. A tight smile. No contact. Where are all the other ex-lovers, now? How destroyed were they? As the writer reads her words about The Tower, she's trying not to cry. I can't tell what the audience is feeling. I can't tell who they're seeing. I can't tell who I'm seeing. I stroke the air, as if that could offer some comfort. But where is comfort needed? With me, or with other people who are far more destroyed than I am?

The audience is quiet. Emotions shrink. Hiding.

The writer finishes with a sob pushed into the last word in her mouth.

The audience clap as she returns to her seat. There is ice in the air between their palms.

Hope approaches the microphone.

I'm staring at Hope's boots again as she speaks her final words. I can tell she's in love, or is about to be. She has a happy secret note hidden inside her voice.

The audience clap for the writers and then they clap for the festival and they clap for tarot cards and finally, they clap for Hope.

Now this event is over I won't have to think about the Three of Swords any more, or the heartbreak it represents. I'm glad I didn't write about a thrice-stabbed heart.

The audience shuffles, ready to move on. Above the nose-line of a mask, one pair of familiar female eyes glance around. No, I'm mistaken. When the eyes meet mine they are cardboard-blank.

The Tower-writer is still upset. Her body sobs without moving. I lean forward, about to ask if I can do anything to help, but she looks at me with such confusion and anger, I back away.

When Z cried, she cried like a child.

Any questions I have are blocked. There's nothing new to be seen or understood.

The cardboard-blank woman comes rushing towards The Tower-writer and hugs her tight. A lover? A friend? No, definitely a lover because their bodies fit to each other's shape like crab claws. They link arms and walk away through the crowds.

'Stay safe,' I whisper at their retreating backs, though these overused words have no strength.

Gone.

Above the chattering audience the air is pale blue and green and white with relief. Voices are talking about how it's great everyone wore masks and kept far enough apart and how lucky we are that these events can happen here at all and how good it is that writers are still writing and that people can, for now, meet other people outside of their houses.

I say goodbye to the other two writers, hug Hope and thank her for gathering us to read. From the glow in her eyes, I'm even more certain she's in love and with someone or something that'll be good for her.

The audience is scattering and everyone's chatting to someone. A grey-brown woman in a red mask frowns and disappears behind an optimistic woman in a polka-dot dress. One of them wants to go dancing. The other one doesn't. They're going to go dancing.

I'm feeling too many things which aren't mine.

The Tower fills my head. It has a ticking clock at the top of it. The clock is painted with Z's face. It cracks and falls. Numbers one to twelve and all the letters of the alphabet scatter across a concrete floor, making new combinations of old and broken things.

All along the mall large groups of people are heading out to pubs, small groups of people are going home. I walk past masks and masks and masks. Conflicting smells. Sweat. Hair product. Blue. Bubblegum vape scent. Lilac. Chips. Purple. Colours trail past in lines of voice-sounds. Red. Green. Yellow. Yellow again. Far-too-bright yellow. The white burst of distant shouts, pink-muffled voices.

Tonight I'm seeing too much because I'm not able to see enough.

I need to be able to see the frown starting in the jaw before it reaches the eyebrows. Whether the eye-expressions match or mis-match the lips. This information is really important—it's how I know who's safe and who's dangerous. Without it, I'm searching for more.

From a group of men, one shouts in my direction, 'What the fuck are you doing?' I can't tell which one shouted, if it's me or someone

154

else he's shouting at. Again. Brown-orange burst of voice, 'I said, what the fuck are you doing?'

I walk faster.

At a bus stop I step through a metal door and am driven away.

On the bus home, I don't feel so great, but I know what to do. I put my headphones on and tune out all the noise. People become shadows as I stare out of the windows at the rush of passing buildings.

When I'm at home I'll do safe and ordinary things, gardening, hoovering, cooking, working, eating, sleeping. But whatever I do, it'll take me a while to stop thinking about The Tower. It's got in too deep. I'll catch myself staring into space, unsure where I've just been.

The other writers didn't notice me and won't remember me at all. And now, I've caught an echo of The Tower. It's brought some jagged fragments of emotions. From then, or now? From the writer, from me, or from Z? It's impossible to know.

Empathy splinters.

Over the next few days, I'll have to try hard to feel the floorboards beneath my feet, to feel Morgan's arms around me, to feel her cheek against my lips and my lips against her cheek, to feel the water of the shower, the smooth texture of the kitchen counter, cat fur against my fingertips.

I'm leaning my forehead against the window on the bus, feeling intense shoulder pain. I'm carrying The Tower home with me in a sack on my shoulders. It is stones against my spine. I want to climb a mountain and drop it in a neat pile at the top, but it's dragging me down to the ground.

The bus pulls up to a bus stop and more people get off than on.

I imagine that Z is surrounded by unbroken walls and strange ornaments, bright-painted furniture and a kind lover who'll take care of her. Someone strong. Someone she won't be able to destroy.

I don't wish her harm, but I can tell from the weight of these stones against my spine, harm is inevitable, for someone.

That's what happens to The Tower.

It destroys itself and everything around it.

Tower to rubble.

Rubble to stone.

Stone to splinter.

Fairweather

Morgan is away for two weeks. I'm trying to remember what it was like when people visited each other or met up socially. But I can't quite connect to these memories. I was trying to make friends here. But then the pandemic happened and I stopped trying. That was probably a bad mistake.

I'm sitting at the table with a coffee and my phone. This is day eleven of not speaking to anyone. I've been enjoying the silence but have just realised that if I got ill or had an accident, there's no one obvious to call.

I don't even know how to answer my phone. It's fairly new. About six months old.

On Facebook, Twitter, Instagram, there are people I haven't heard from in a very long time. I wonder if they are also looking at lists of people on their phone and thinking they haven't heard from any of these people for a long time.

Maybe the phone is a problem.

I think everyone I love is on it and is easily available. I think I am easily available to them. I can falsely believe that I live in a crowd of people who know each other well. But there's been no one apart from me inside this house for the past eleven days. My fingertips touch images of my friends in sequences of taps and swipes.

Phone communication is two-dimensional. Unicode limits the characters. Text is predicted and predictable. 2D faces are an illusion of three-dimensions. Emojis simplify complex emotions into likes / loves / care / sad / angry... But surely emotions are three-dimensional? Breadth, height and depth. There are 3D people I've met here in Wellington who aren't on social media, so they aren't flattened like the 2D friends who live inside this phone.

I'm thinking of the 3D creative writing tutor who offered to go for a walk with me.

And of my 3D ex-student who lives down the road from here. We went for a drink together once.

I'm thinking of a 3D art lecturer I met when I was doing my

PhD. B was more like a rabbit than a human. She and I went for a drink in central Wellington because she'd read and liked my writing. We found a quiet corner and drank wine and talked about art and writing and animals and introverts and nature. B seemed familiar, a feeling I treasured. At the end of the night she hopped away along rain-damp pavements, waving goodbyes at me, promising to see me again. I called back, laughing, 'Yes, let's do that!'

Outside, a storm is coming.

We didn't go for another drink.

The fourth dimension is time. We didn't become 4D friends.

The next time I saw B was by chance, in a corridor at work. She said, 'We were going to be friends, I could tell. But you disappeared.'

I frowned down at her shiny shoes, thinking that rabbits probably find footwear quite uncomfortable. I replied, 'But I didn't disappear. Not this time. I've stayed.'

'Let's email each other,' she said. 'Try again.' She smiled at me, nose twitching slightly.

I grinned. 'I'd like that.'

But neither of us have emailed. Perhaps it's the pandemic. No one wants to make new friends right now. I don't want to risk catching Covid and passing it to Morgan. She's terrified of catching it as she thinks she'll die. Perhaps it's never easy to begin new friendships as we get older, for some of us. Someone who's more rabbit than human is probably as awkward as I am.

The last time I saw B we were both on the same panel at a conference. She had a bag of costume accessories with her, made of recycled furs and soft fabrics. She offered them to all the panellists to dress up in. She put on a pair of tall ears and looked perfectly rabbity. None of the other panellists took her up on her offer. I took a fur lined muff from her bag, sunk my hands inside it and stroked the soft fur. It kept me calm as I waited for my turn to read.

Large drops of rain land and slide down the window as I sip the last of my cold coffee.

Maybe I'll try harder to see B again when this latest Covid wave has passed through.

It's strange to be in Wellington without Morgan. I can feel invisible red threads between us, stretching, linking us. For a moment I close my eyes and find her. She's asleep. I stroke her hair before returning to empty my coffee mug.

Z to A. A to Z. I scroll through Facebook 'friend lists' on my phone. A to Z. Z to A. There's not really anyone it feels natural or right to contact if I get lonelier than I can cope with. People would find it odd because it's never happened before, me getting in touch and saying I'd like a chat. Is that selfish? Should I send messages to other people and ask them if they'd like a chat? I seem to have forgotten how to begin new conversations, or resume old ones.

It must be the same for everyone across the whole world, right now. Friendships have changed, even for people who live within the same geographical areas. People are divided in terms of opinions and beliefs, reactions and fears and also resilience. Some of us feel stronger. Some of us feel diminished. Five stages of grief, in no particular order: denial, anger, bargaining, depression, acceptance.[5] We haven't yet had the chance to talk about this. To understand what's happened to us all.

Three sparrows are on the empty washing line, interspersed by my second-favourite pegs—the bright ones with a slit on the top and bottom.

The sparrows watch me through the window. I can hear them saying:

> *There are no real friends*
> *in that shiny block in your hand.*

No, it is a shiny phone full of friends.
It's where all my flattened friends live now, in 2D.
My world has changed.
No, the whole world has changed.
Has your world changed? (Who am I talking to?)
I'm silently watching them all—the friends I used to be right beside.

A loves B with the heart emoji
followed by C, D the fun-we-had with E's smily face emoji
denial

---

5   Elisabeth Kübler-Ross, 1969.

followed by an FGHIJK impromptu Zoom party with L's cocktail
glass emoji,
followed by M, N, O worriers is-everything-OK-thumbs-up emoji
denial, bargaining
(guilt-have-we-all-over-indulged?) P, Q, R, S's interruption
of T's soggy batman and U and V's lost kitten and
denial, bargaining, depression
ooh. Conspiracy theory. Does T mean it?
denial, bargaining, depression, anger
Unfriend/tell off/SHOUT/be gentle to T because of mis-irony or
mis-information
or mis-direction or mis-trust or mis-truth.
denial, bargaining, depression, anger, acceptance...

> *There are no real friends*
> *in that shiny block in your hand.*

I know. But I'm watching
a random stone rolling off a random horse and falling into a random
boat
where is that boat going to? Somewhere the borders are open
wow, W's new shoes. Nice blue, but where are they shipped from?
U posts yet another photograph of food in brown-red colours and
slime-texture.
Look away. Clag-flavours. Unfriend U? Too harsh.
I like this picture of lichen but how did I meet the person who
posted it
will it be too strange for them if I comment because they don't
remember either?
I don't remember ever talking to U and do I really know an X?
Y has Covid. Y sends a hug-emoji, for care, to Z. Z has Covid. Not
that Z. Another Z.
I'm not sure how to interrupt but I must have said something
I've been sat here for over two hours. I haven't
interrupted / is this depression or acceptance
no, I haven't said anything at all.
I've just been watching flattened people for two 2D hours
my attention span is getting shorter.

There are no real friends
in that shiny block in your hand.

No, it is a shiny phone full of people.
It's a lovely little place where all my friends live, now.
I used to be far lonelier than this.

Did you?

Didn't I?
Once upon a time I invented a list of new words for different kinds
of loneliness.
That was long before the pandemic, before migration.
I miss robins. Their flashes of red. I've never seen one here.
I'm so used to being lonely, now. I can barely even feel it.

Then why aren't you smiling?

I send another care emoji to A, B, C, D, E, F, G, H, I, J...
because they have all got Covid.
Real friends speak in likes-and-care-and-love emoji. I like their likes.
Real friends, liking each other right now.
Not the ones who only exist in memories
or the friends in this city I haven't tried hard enough to get to know.

Robins fight to the death.
They wouldn't be welcomed here.
When we don't want to fight
we get all blissed-upwards—
kissing the clouds.

The rain has stopped. The sky is darkening again.
It's almost night-black unless I'm here on this phone,
and there is screen light and so many people
(my attention span is frazzled—
need to slow my head down and read a book instead)
but unless I say something, none of them talk back.

I don't feel like saying much right now.
I'm wrapped in my own invisible wings.
Self-contained in this silence.
Telling myself solitude has always been the safest place.

Remember that nursery rhyme?
Poor things, poor things.
Hide your head under a wing.

The phone is the problem.
I put down the phone
and leave all my alphabetical
friends on the table.

In the garden, the sparrows and I wait for a storm.
The air tightens.
Small brown birds are perched everywhere.
Claws tight-grip lines, wires, branches, gutters.

A rumble. Darkening.
The air breaks.
The sparrows fall silent as ghosts
and disappear.

Rain slashes down.
I'm smiling the rain into my mouth.
Those flighty sparrows,
gone again, like a dream switched off.

Fair weatherers.

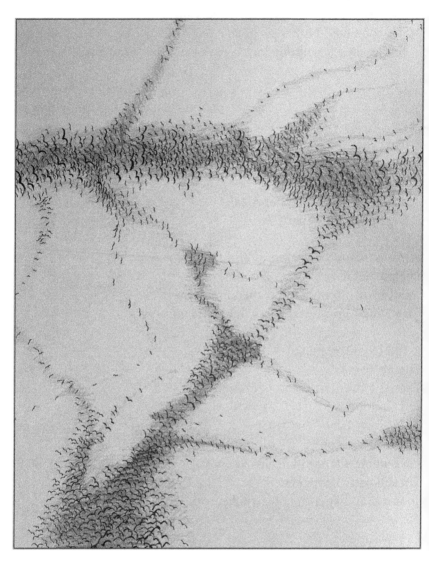

Flock of Ghosts III

Ten Words for Loneliness

Despane– The loneliness of feeling misunderstood, unloved or unheard by someone who used to understand, love or listen.

Starn– Craving something or someone to be there but knowing it's/they're not. Wanting to bite something.

Youache– Where a specific person is missed and only their physical presence will cure the ache of missing them.

Ignornly– The kind of loneliness that other people notice, but don't mention to the person they think is lonely. Their expression shows sympathy, but also a little wariness, as if loneliness could be contagious.

Solilone– A type of melancholia experienced while gazing at a wide-skied landscape. A longing for strangeness, for the unreal or the surreal to appear.

Idealone– A hankering for an imagined scenario—where it's the idea of the situation that causes the loneliness. For example, the 'ideal' of the perfect friend sitting opposite on the sofa, laughing over wine and confessions and saying all of the right things.

Achiposs– The ache of missing out on experiencing something beautiful, because it is impossible.

Disampty– Where the immediate environment is problematic – usually in practical ways. The rubbish split all over the floor, the smoke alarm is going off, work is waiting, the clock is ticking, the umbrella's broken, it's lashing with rain and there's no one else around.

Crowdsad– Felt while around many other people. Crying while walking along streets crammed with strangers, feeling unable to speak during a burbling conversation in which others are talking loudly and not leaving any gaps.

Feartrap– when alone, overactive fears producing images of other people becoming monstrous.

Dreams of Birds and Ghosts

I

After half-reading a bird book[6], the words come loose from the pages and flit around my mind. I close my eyes and enter a desolate dream-scene. On a solitary alder tree, the birds seem lost—they perch on gale-spared branches, pointing their beaks into the air.

The tree is croaking so I ask the tree, 'Are you my dad?'

There's a lightning crack and something shrieks,

Call a Whoever-bird—nasty speaking.

In a nightmare, the Panic-bird wakes from a hole in the ground and sees a feathered man. His ghostly form is disfigured by a swirl of scorched leaves.

Pecking at air, the Panic-bird asks,

What are you?

'I'm a fallen bird.' The man blinks and disappears.

All around me it is winter.

Snow falls.

I am inside a ghost's dream of moulting feathers.

II

I don't know where Bird-ghosts live or die. I am hunting my dad's ghost without weapons, without directions, without a map.

I am moving further away from my real body. I am many bodies. I am searching many bodies, for his ghost. Wanting to believe in possession. Wanting to possess.

In this dream I am a country with farmlands and big gardens, the Sparrow-ghost flies fast and close to my ground.

---

6   Aristophanes, *The Birds*. Some of the words in this section are from this play.

Crows croak, shouting about shame.

And I am soil, trying to tell a Bird-ghost some old story about: noise bang rock, head stone and knock.

Air flows upwards for so long I can't speak at all. And now I am a Stitchbird.

Spread both feet, spend chirp upon chirp, singing back at the Crows about shame.

If my father was here, he would listen. No one is listening, so he is not here.

III

As an endangered Stitchbird, I have trouble calling, 'Keep your distance.'

I am in New Zealand weaving silence from threads. Stories and pictures and words which won't ever be spoken. I weave tired secrets as grey threads and dusty webs. When there is no one else around who remembers the past, we can make ourselves up. Our stories are misplaced, cut loose from all kinds of threads that bind us together.

I go to a second-hand shop and buy six handkerchiefs, half-embroidered by someone else's grandmother. Interrupted by death, or disinterest. I have so few objects from my own past, with memories attached to them. The threads of these handkerchiefs are old. A half-finished leaf, stitched in the corner. I pretend these handkerchiefs are significant and belong to me.

Thumbing their fabric, I conjure an image of my paternal grandmother sewing. A net curtain moving as a breeze came in through her open window. From outside, the song of thrushes. The smell of peaches. A later memory of both of us stitching name-tags into the seams of her knickers when she was about to move into a care home. Sunlight moves across green embroidery threads.

The handkerchiefs are so dusty they no longer shine but for now I love them for pretending to contain my memories.

A ghost changes nature, becomes a Claw-bird and flies all the way here. It asks of me, soft,

Are you lonely?

'No, no, no.' Too soft turns hard-quick when too soft is a lie.

What's the truth?

'I've always been lonely because I've always felt like an odd girl and still do.' Middle-child girl with three brothers. Vegetarian English family living in rural Scotland in the seventies and eighties. Only interested in art and writing. Terrible at even basic maths. Lesbian. Hypersensitive to sounds, emotions, movement beneath pavements, change and distance.

This Claw-bird is not my father's ghost. It is here to unsettle me.
Falling silent it tilts its head, eyeing me.
The distance it has flown to ask me to tell the truth is overwhelming.
The Claw-bird flurries away.
My dad has never been here in New Zealand
his memories don't exist here,
so what if his ghost can never come and find me here?
I can't I couldn't I can't
think these thoughts when I'm fully awake
I can't I couldn't I can't
speak for crying.

IV

I keep stitching. I always keep stitching. White threads to a bed, a pillow to my head, my head threads a hair-width, to stitch my eyes closed, stitch my own lips.

Stitch myself silent into an embroidered body made from thread-feathers.

Habitation, fence it with walls—evolve as a trap-and-net bird.

V

Twirl clouds and sky over seascape. I am testing my own limits. A flight across the whole planet.

You fly beneath me, Ghost-gull, as white wings over grey waves. You touch and don't touch foam. You're crying out with love for the of the sea.

The Ghost-gull kisses and kisses and kisses wave-spray away, under a reflected moon.

Falling, I land against silver rocks. Alone on a strange shore, I curse the exhaustion of flight-restrictions. I bite against these rocks.

This is a landscape of permanent wingache.

VI

Dreams of birds and ghosts merge together. They slump like pillow-trapped feathers.

The Little-ghost, unlike other ghosts, dreams at twilight. It cries when it is on the ground. The Little-ghost can't hop, but runs quite fast. People dislike it.

The Reed-ghosts live nearby, dreaming near ponds, flying only short distances. Their song is thin.

Enigmatic Maggle-ghosts have nest ambitions. Hidden deep inside their throats, dark ink spreads. When threatened, they spit out unspoken words.

The Butcher-ghost is beautiful and fierce—it has nightmares and impales its kill on thornbushes.

Shrieking like a Howl owl, ghosts and their dreams are everywhere.

He is none of these Bird-ghosts. Dream creatures.

Half-here, half-there.

Even disguised, I would recognise him anywhere.

VII

Glutton, another glutton.

Peck peck peck.

The longer I'm trapped in any dream of distances and attempts to fly, the more I understand that birds and ghosts are everywhere.

How lonely does the sky feel?

Ghosts come from the edges and spread upwards into mid-air colonies. Rage-emissions.

Green-ghosts flurry away.

VIII

I'm tired so I find a path to walk along. Tall grasses, rhododendron bushes, gorse out-of-place.

Is he anywhere in these half-way places? Under that root? Is he those yellow flowers? Is he a grub, lichen, a moth? Is there such a thing as a Moth-ghost?

When a Moth-ghost finally appears, I hold out cupped hands, offering it torn grass-threads.

It chirrups and snatches my unstitches for future nesting.

IX

With no threads left to stitch with, I seek out watery places.

The Come-hither birds snap up lake water.

His ghost is not here. His ghost is not in a half-way place. His ghost is only there.

I have to travel further, for longer.

I have to forget dreams, but still remember their meanings.

In this dream I am almost gone.

Beside the shore an albatross flits over lapping waves.

Come-hither.

X

All the birds fly wide,

whoop and whoop!

The fear I haven't mentioned, I don't dare to mention it.

Time is not linear. Not to ghosts and not to those who are seeking them.

(How far is too far? How long is too long? Are time and distance, breakable?)

Fear is sprung. A trap-in-the-mind.

The only cure for wingache is to spread dreams of wings towards the far north,

north of the winter

as part of a vast flock of ghosts.

2020
Big Talk

How long have you been living here?

I don't know. Six, maybe five and a half, maybe three years.

Why don't you know how long you've been living here for?

Because it doesn't matter how long.

How short have you been living here?

I don't know. Six, maybe five and a half, maybe two years.

Why don't you know how short you've been living here for?

Because it doesn't matter.

How high or low have you been since you've been living here?

I don't know. Six, maybe five and a half, maybe four times my armspan and weight.

Why don't you know how high or low you've been?

It doesn't matter.

You don't like small talk.

It makes me feel like a lonely ghost.
Time and distance don't seem important to ghosts.
Six, maybe five and a half, maybe three times more loneliness.

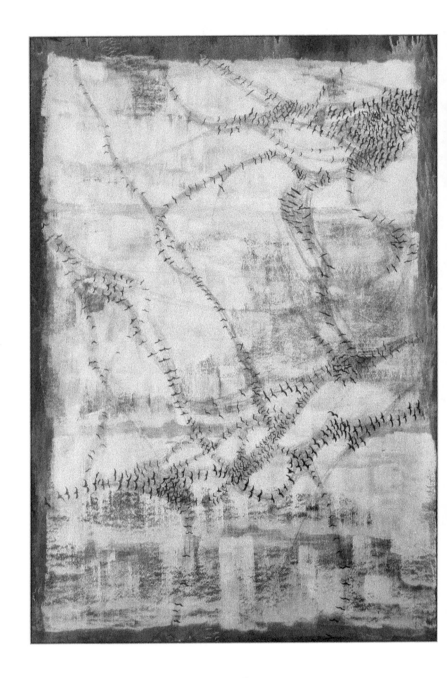

Flock of Ghosts IV

172

Eleven Words for Loneliness

Despane– The loneliness of feeling misunderstood, unloved or unheard by someone who used to understand, love or listen.

Starn– Craving something or someone to be there but knowing it's/ they're not. Wanting to bite something.

Youache– Where a specific person is missed and only their physical presence will cure the ache of missing them.

Ignornly– The kind of loneliness that other people notice, but don't mention to the person they think is lonely. Their expression shows sympathy, but also a little wariness, as if loneliness could be contagious.

Solilone– A type of melancholia experienced while gazing at a wide-skied landscape. A longing for strangeness, for the unreal or the surreal to appear.

Idealone– A hankering for an imagined scenario—where it's the idea of the situation that causes the loneliness. For example, the 'ideal' of the perfect friend sitting opposite on the sofa, laughing over wine and confessions and saying all of the right things.

Achiposs– The ache of missing out on experiencing something beautiful, because it is impossible.

Disampty– Where the immediate environment is problematic – usually in practical ways. The rubbish split all over the floor, the smoke alarm is going off, work is waiting, the clock is ticking, the umbrella's broken, it's lashing with rain and there's no one else around.

Crowdsad– Felt while around many other people. Crying while walking along streets crammed with strangers, feeling unable to speak during a burbling conversation in which others are talking loudly and not leaving any gaps.

Feartrap– when alone, overactive fears producing images of other people becoming monstrous.

Priclash– Keeping emotions or secrets private while desperately wanting to let them out.

Lonely Ghosts

I

Living people are made up of millions of layers.

Throughout a human lifespan, many of these layers peel off or are ripped away.

These layers become lonely ghosts.

The living leave their ghosts lying around everywhere.

II

I was seventeen when one of my loneliest ghosts was made. I like to think there was an ominous sign that night. Something I missed. A raven falling from the sky, perhaps. Dropping to the ground at my feet like a shadow ripped from a cloud. Something inexplicable.

But really, there was no warning. It was just another ordinary Friday night.

In Scotland, a man is pinning someone down against concrete in a primary school playground. That someone looks like me, aged seventeen. She looks at the stars with desperation in her eyes, like they will fall and cut him to shreds, like they will shout or scream for help, like they will protect her.

But the stars are only holes in the sky.

I drift in and out of them, threading myself thin.

Seen from this angle, the man is raping someone else.

She raises her head, strains, and slams it against concrete.

Blank.

When she opens her eyes again, I'm back.

He's saying, 'Sorry sorry sorry. Stop crying. Sorry, stop crying.' He tries to smudge my mascara tears away and smears my own blood across my face.

'Oh god,' he says. 'Oh god.'

Staring at him, I'm thinking he might kill me. Staring at him, I'm thinking I don't mind the idea of death too much. Staring at him, I'm surprised about my lack of fear.

I say, 'I just need to get to a phone. To call a taxi home.'

I leave my ghost in that playground so I can get home and have a bath with the door locked and my hands closing my ears, closing my eyes, hands rubbing soap with no scent to it, washing away blood. So I can keep my bruises hidden. So I can still leave home as planned and go to art college in Carlisle just before my eighteenth birthday.

III

Small ghosts haunt a windy garden in southwest Scotland. This is a garden in which songs are sung to daisies, a garden which peapods are stolen from. This is a garden which scratches and stings my three brothers and me as we tear through weeds as crownless kings wearing towels-for-capes.

This garden contains a deep ditch our parents are afraid the smallest of us will drown in. A ditch, which, knowing they are afraid, we constantly bury ourselves in. We are four small corpses in this ditch at the end of every holiday just before, six miles away, the primary school gates open again.

This garden is a garden that can't stop the year turning and drawing us back to a school filled with bullies who hate the kinds of crownless children who'd bury themselves in a ditch in an overgrown garden.

At the end of every summer, four small ghosts haunt the ditch in a windy garden in south west Scotland. It's dank and muddy inside the ditch. It's hidden beneath brambles and tangled nettles, like a trench dug for war.

IV

One of my ghosts lives in France, in the kitchen of someone else's house. They live there just because there is a dishwasher. My ghost crouches on the tiled kitchen floor, listening to the gurgles of plates being washed. It claps its transparent hands because the dishwasher sounds like a waterfall.

V

In England, one of my ghosts is haunting a bus-stop in Carlisle. The bus-stop is near enough to the station for predatory men to arrive, assault women, and leave undetected. The bus-stop is where young art students wait for buses to take them back to some lodging room across town. The ghost I've left in Carlisle is an eighteen-year-old who feels as ancient as the stones of Hadrian's wall. She wears parrot-feathers plaited through her long hair and a torn frock coat tightly buttoned from boots to neck. This eighteen-year-old ghost who feels as ancient as stones knows no one in this town. She doesn't eat, doesn't sleep and never blinks. Her lace-gloved hands are hidden in deep pockets.

She haunts the bus stop, waiting for a tall man in a clean trench coat and shiny shoes who is there exactly an hour after dusk in the Autumn of 1989.

Clenched in her right hand, hidden deep in a pocket, is a silver flick-knife.

'Touch me again,' she whispers, though no one is listening.

VI

One of my ghosts is on her first ever plane flight, from Gatwick to Glasgow. The plane rises through clouds and beyond into pure light. The intensifying force of the engines make her feel like she has doubled in size and is side-by-side with her own imaginary twin as they stare through the curved window, soaking all the light and moist textures of clouds into all four of their eyes. They would be so joyful if this breathless bright moment marked the end of ground-bound living. If they died right now in this extraordinary overcloud place, they wouldn't mind at all.

VII

Our neighbours in Wellington are so glad they'll be seeing their family for a birthday party this weekend—they all live further north. 'It's been two months,' they say to us over the garden fence. 'Ages.'

There's yet another wave of the virus hitting the UK and the government aren't even telling people to wear masks any more. Morgan's youngest brother has Covid. My middle brother has Covid.

'We're so lucky,' our neighbours say.

We are not living the same lives as our neighbours in New Zealand.

'We're learning to live with it,' our brothers say.

We are not living the same lives as our families in the UK.

But if Morgan and I are living like ghosts, at least we are ghosts together.

VIII

In Brighton I am unhappy for too many years. I can't remember what I do or don't like any more. But I have a special power—I can walk through the busy streets of Brighton crying or laughing or sighing, and be completely invisible. Being invisible in a crowd creates many ghosts. They peel off my body like unwanted feathers. I feel each one of my ghosts fall. I step over them and keep walking, pale feathers scattering along the pavement behind me.

One day I hear ambulance sirens and am convinced it is me, this one, the one who keeps walking, who is the ghost.

My *living* body must therefore be lying behind me on the pavement. I've managed to step out of it and walk away. The ambulance is coming to take it to the hospital or the morgue, whichever is needed. I imagine strangers surrounding my body, making phone calls, searching my wrists and neck for pulses of life.

IX

Five people sit separately along the pavement outside a supermarket in Wellington. Begging bowl, begging hat, begging cardboard letter, cupped hand, an unstrummed guitar. It's winter. Woollen hat. Thick scarf. A dog-in-a-blanket. Gloves. It is Friday. 5.00pm. Home-time. Weekend-time. End of work-time.

Working-ghosts stride past the five people begging on the pavement, rushing to get to the supermarket, to get home. Working-ghosts carry phones that shine screen light on their faces.

Five beggars today. Yesterday at the same hour, there were three.

Working-ghosts rush past the five people begging on the pavement, as if fearful about why there are so many more and so quickly.

Pigeons perch on the supermarket gutter, watching all the ghosts in the street below. I stand in a doorway opposite the supermarket, watching the pigeons I shared my lunch with yesterday.

Working-ghosts are afraid. They're afraid of people who ask them for money. They're afraid of winter, of joblessness, of the coldness of the pavement.

X

I've left one of my ghosts sitting on the doorstep of an empty cottage at Kintyre which I was living in while working as a caretaker for five alone-months. My ghost sits on the doorstep wrapped in a blanket watching V-shaped trails of geese cross a white winter sky.

This ghost is a Waiting-ghost. It knows something is about to change.

Soon, it will love someone.

Soon, it will be loved.

And when these two things happen at the same time, this ghost will transform into something that understands how to be alive.

XI

Leaving a home-trap is far easier than I thought it would be:

Get rid of any possessions that can't fit in a rucksack. Switch off all digital communication and walk away as quickly as possible.

The ghost who would have stayed in the home-trap remains there as a left-behind thing, as a thinning twirl of hair, as a rusted razor blade, as a silent gasp of realisation that still hangs in the air.

Head towards wherever the coldest air is coming from. Stop in a place where there are no more people. No more wires cutting through the sky. No more poles, holding up the wires. A bare wide sky over a gorse-soaked moor. Rocks. Bleached bones. Part of a spine.

It is possible to see the whole horizon, all the way to the edge.

And it is possible to do the one thing ghosts can't do—breathe.

XII

My seventeen-year-old ghost still haunts the playground in Scotland. She's stuck there, rocking herself on the swings. At night-time she lies on the slide and tells the stars they are only holes in the sky.

All these years later, the primary school now has high wire fences all around its playground. The fence keeps children caged-in during the days and it keeps violent men caged-out during the nights.

Ravens land on the wire fence like shadows and torment my ghost by showing her their natural weapons:

> *Look, knife-beak.*
> *Look, stab-claws.*
> *Claw craw craw!*

Each dusk my seventeen-year-old ghost walks slowly around the inside of the fence as if it is a cage. She waits for starholes to appear, thrumming the wire with transparent fingertips.

She tells herself that every night is just another ordinary Friday night.

Sometimes she hears the shriek of a falling raven but she tells herself there's nothing there but shadows.

On one ordinary Friday night, she'll tell the ravens, 'I wish I could grow wings.'

On another ordinary Friday night, she will.

XIII

Ghosts are made up of millions of layers.

Throughout a ghost's existence, many of these layers peel off or are ripped away.

These layers become birds.

Ghosts that have become birds fly around everywhere.

Wingache

I've been hunting for childhood memories. This is partly because I've recently started the long process of having an autism spectrum assessment and many unanswerable questions have been asked. It's also because I'm in New Zealand with the borders closed and my relatives are all in Scotland. I have memories of family photographs, but no photographs. When I try to make sense of things which aren't fully remembered, I think of stories I've been told by other family members and memories of photographic images. I think of the cells in my body and their distance from familiar people's cells. I think of the dull ache in my shoulder blades.

There's a torn photograph album in my mum's house that our family used to occasionally look at together. It contains a square photo of me aged about three, standing on the wobbly stool cleaning my dad's rusty car. I can't remember doing this, so I probably didn't fall. There's another photo of me perched on my mum's knees in my great-grandad's garden, laughing at the bubbles she's blowing like they're made of magic. I can't remember this moment, either. This photo is my mum's memory, of her lilac-coloured clothes and of me grinning up at her. There's another photo of me gazing at giant carthorses in the field near my Auntie's wedding—I don't remember this but can imagine noticing the heavy bones of their muscular shoulders, the fur at their ankles, their clomping hooves.

There's also a close-up photo of my black and white eye. This one does have a memory attached—of looking for my dad inside a camera lens. Of trying to make him see me.

I've never met anyone who remembers being born. We rely on our parents to tell us about it. According to my mum, I was born 'feeling sound'. My eyes were bright and my hands moved strangely. A slow flowing motion. 'Graceful,' she's always told me. 'Like you were stroking the movement of our voices in the air. Your hands were the first thing I noticed about you.'

I have no memory of this. The memories I have of the torn photograph album are fading. I wonder now if I was born feeling sounds, or feeling the movements of air. If it was air, my most vivid memories, beyond flat photographs, beyond familial stories, make slightly more sense. The ache in my shoulder blades I still feel now, makes sense.

When I was a baby, I could fly.

The strongest memories I have, are of flying. I'd extend my arms, reaching up. The whole sky swooped down, picked me up and carried me as high as I wanted to go. A rush of air beneath me, filling my arms and chest—my arm-span was far wider than my fingertips. As a baby I flew above the clouds. I'd get blown around up there. Colours. Light. Temperature. My ability to fly continued while I slowly learned to walk.

Once I was walking, I'd leap into flight, but I could only fly just beneath the clouds. I hovered in and out of them taking mouthfuls of moist air, watching the landscape below.

Flying was not breath-less, but breath-more. Air was noisy, rhythmic, blustering, whistling. It was part of the body and all through the body. Air itself was a vast body, containing many smaller bodies—of clouds, birds, aeroplanes, hang-gliders, hot-air-balloons. Raindrops, insects, snowflakes, dust, hail. There could easily have been many other flying babies all around me in the clouds, though like me, they were invisible.

Flying felt like this:

I leap a short distance and am lifted upwards as the air thins. In the sky I'm overpowered by gusts, part of everything and nothing at the same time. Silent laughter moves carelessly from my scalp to my toenails. Every cell in my body is intensely alive. The height and direction of flight is chosen by making tiny adjustments within the muscles of the shoulder blades and the angles of the outstretched arms. How small I feel, up here where clouds and sunlight and moonlight are all part of a different conversation. How big I feel, as if the body extends so much further than its skin-edges. Twist one way and the other. Drift. Rise or fall, it doesn't matter. Nothing matters apart from breath and these changes of temperature and rushes of moving air. Fly lower—the body weighs more as it drops. Fly higher, become lighter, there's more air movement, less control.

White seabirds circle over a thick ocean. Along the coast, stone-lines divide fields. There's a trail of lamp-eyed coaches moving towards distant cities. A snaking train. Witch-hat spires and curved domes. Tiles and moss, a circular dovecot with a flurry of white feathers in the grass. The tin roof of a barn. Home is here—these chimneys on an oblong grey roof, field-surrounded, tangles of hawthorn, gorse and fuchsia. Swerve to avoid the gutters. Skirt along the dipped washing line like it's a broken tightrope, toes hitting pegs. Dropping, there's soaked grass, a thud to the soles, weight, solid ground.

Land.

The heights I could fly to dropped as I reached three years old. I could just about make it up to church-height when I was four. Then telegraph-wire-height. Then house-height. Heavy-carthorse-height. Father-mother-height. Age five. Brother-height. Grass-height. I could still feel air under my arms, carrying me along just above the ground. Then nothing. A leap. A thud. Another leap. Another thud.

The longer I spent walking on the ground, the harder it became to fly away from it.

Our rented stone home was an old schoolhouse on a peninsula in southwest Scotland. The windiest place in the UK. My mum had the radio on constantly in our kitchen full of baking smells, drying laundry and cats. It was the only warm room. Whenever a gale-force warning was announced on the radio I'd slip away and thrust my feet into welly boots. Morning or night, I'd rush outside into the garden. Near the washing line there was a small downwards slope. Red dressing-gown flapping, I'd run building momentum, arms outstretched, and leap. Each time I'd land awkwardly on my heavy feet.

At eight years old I remember hugging myself, knees to chest in wet grass. A gale blustered around me, sleet pinch-punching my shoulder blades, gusts knotting my tangled hair. Gazing upwards, soak-faced, I finally accepted I wouldn't fly again. I knew how much heavier and duller everything would become and how quickly. High above me clouds as heavy as carthorses charged in rhythmic circles across the brightening, darkening, brightening sky.

These memories are confusing, because they aren't logical. And yet they're more vivid than all my other childhood memories. It's entirely possible I can't fully distinguish between dreams, imagination and memory. But I can't be the only person who could fly when they were a baby. Perhaps we all try to forget the memories which don't make logical sense.

Memories which involve the parts of our bodies which remember, cell deep.

The parts of our bodies that ache.

This memory lives in my shoulder blades as a dull wingache. It aches hardest whenever I feel trapped.

If a baby is born touching sounds in the air and with the ability to fly, is the baby part human, part bird, part ghost, before it becomes a child?

Unbroken

There are cracks in these white walls   that the last earthquake made. There's a plant growing in through the windowframe, tiny green   leaves carrying drops of dampness from exterior to interior. Through the window sunshine appears   and so strangely, brings rain. The sunshine and the rain are both gone so quickly, it's as if they   weren't really there at all. There's a bird, a pīwakawaka that's out the back when I'm looking   out of the back window and it flies around the front when I'm looking out of the front window.   This pīwakawaka has a fan tail, it flips and flups it around, back forth back, dancing with   air. The pīwakawaka is a messenger between the living and the dead. The three slate clocks I   made in Scotland have batteries from back then and the batteries have rusted and run brown   lines down this white wall in New Zealand. New Zealand is where Morgan and I   love and live and love. Outside in our back garden the neighbour's bright-eyed cat has left   a disembowelled rat on the grass. Heavy flies crawl around the deep red jewels of its organs.   On the garden path among fallen rose petals there's a dead wētā, legs-up, yellow articulated   body in a curve, angular legs folded over and over and under and under themselves. My   father is buried in Scotland and an alder tree marks his grave. I am under a kōwhai tree in   New Zealand, standing on blood-soaked grass and thinking about there being so many   dead things around our home today. Thinking about there being so many deaths in every country.   This country was for a while so enviably safe. We were safe in our houses. We were as   safe as our earthquake-cracked houses. Morgan's mother Jeanette died of Covid-19 in   January and just before we watched her funeral on a laptop, a blackbird flew into our home   to look at all the bright flowers which had been delivered for Morgan. We had been watching   the news from other countries there was not enough oxygen and not enough vaccine and   in the countries that most needed it, the vaccine wasn't getting through fast enough.   In Scotland it is my mother's birthday today and she had her second vaccine two weeks   ago. The numbers of deaths are rising and rising and rising with each sunfall and sunfall   and sunfall. The whole sky is closed to our unvaccinated and vaccinated bodies, there is no   way to reach out, to help, to mend, to say, here, take my oxygen, this swirl of breath from my   self-isolated lungs, take anything I have in my airways, in my guts, in my bones, if there's   anything I have which will help. For a long while we were too lucky here in New Zealand,   even those of us whose entire families live in other countries, families we still grieve and cry   and hope and long for. Take this too-lucky breath from my self-isolated lungs, take anything   lucky that will help, take these lucky hands, take the lucky silence of this room with   no ticking clocks. Take this pīwakawaka because it is made of magic and let it carry a   message from the living to the dead and from the dead to the living. Let the magic bird tell   all the dead that every organ in their bodies was a precious jewel and that they once had   eyes brighter than the eyes of a hunting cat and candles are still lit for them and fires still   burn for them and trees still grow for them. Tell them even though they have no breath,   plants keep growing through walls even when all of the clocks have stopped. Tell them the   earth they walked on is still alive with its earthquakes and its tree-marked graves and cloud-full   skies and heavy flies. Let the magic bird carry this message to anyone living who needs to hear it: *hold on.* Hold on to love and life and love—hold on like you are the very last tiny green   leaf, carrying the very last raindrop. Hold on, knowing that one day rain will fall again, so   strangely, when the sun finally arrives.

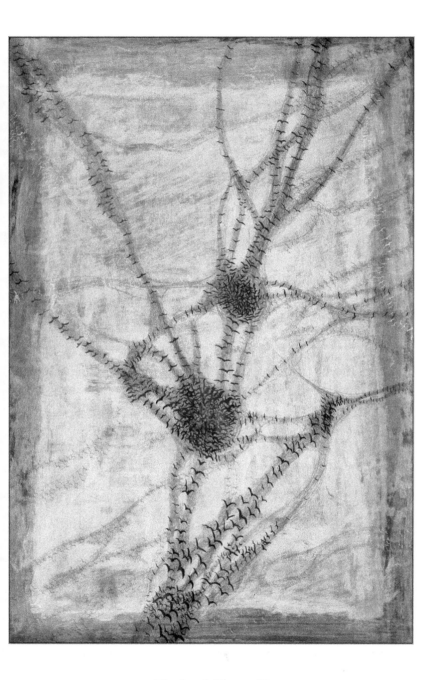

Flock of Ghosts V

Twelve Words for Loneliness

Despane– The loneliness of feeling misunderstood, unloved or unheard by someone who used to understand, love or listen.

Starn– Craving something or someone to be there but knowing it's/they're not. Wanting to bite something.

Youache– Where a specific person is missed and only their physical presence will cure the ache of missing them.

Ignornly– The kind of loneliness that other people notice, but don't mention to the person they think is lonely. Their expression shows sympathy, but also a little wariness, as if loneliness could be contagious.

Solilone– A type of melancholia experienced while gazing at a wide-skied landscape. A longing for strangeness, for the unreal or the surreal to appear.

Idealone– A hankering for an imagined scenario—where it's the idea of the situation that causes the loneliness. For example, the 'ideal' of the perfect friend sitting opposite on the sofa, laughing over wine and confessions and saying all of the right things.

Achiposs– The ache of missing out on experiencing something beautiful, because it is impossible.

Disampty– Where the immediate environment is problematic – usually in practical ways. The rubbish split all over the floor, the smoke alarm is going off, work is waiting, the clock is ticking, the umbrella's broken, it's lashing with rain and there's no one else around.

Crowdsad– Felt while around many other people. Crying while walking along streets crammed with strangers, feeling unable to speak during a burbling conversation in which others are talking loudly and not leaving any gaps.

Feartrap– when alone, overactive fears producing images of other people becoming monstrous.

Priclash– Keeping emotions or secrets private while desperately wanting to let them out.

Xiley– The loneliness of ears: usually during unexpected silence. For example, when any music player suddenly ceases to work and refuses to be fixed.

Sleeping Beauty

You are not here. This white bedroom is usually a sanctuary, for both of us. Only room enough for a bed and a corner bookshelf. The walls, filled with small paintings. My ink drawings of birds hang on the wall above our heads.

But today it's not comforting because we're both in bed while I wake but you are not here. You are asleep, but you've gone far further away than sleep usually takes you to. It's easy enough to see this, from the outside. For the last half-hour since I woke, I've been watching your lips for dreamed-speech, your nostrils for their in-and-exhale and your forehead for the tiny movements that usually reveal your attention is on a dream.

I've whispered, 'Hey, you.'

But no part of you stirs or murmurs a reply.

Beneath our brown linen duvet air fills and empties your lungs. I'm imagining blood spreading warmth through your heart. I'm half-seeing miniature ink-birds flying over our heads beneath the paper lampshade.

Your eyes are not even flickering beneath their lids.

You are submerged in grief for your mother and two of your dearest friends who have recently died. Today you might be unable to wake easily into this world. If there was an earthquake, you might have to jolt awake. But there is only me and this quiet day.

I've seen birds freeze when threatened, glass-eyed, their whole bodies paused for a while. Thanatosis. They disappear from themselves till danger has passed. And when they're safe again they move back into themselves as if they were never really gone at all. I doubt the birds remember what it felt like to be gone; to shift out of themselves and back in again.

You are frightened of Covid, perhaps more than most because of medical issues which make you vulnerable. Covid also exacerbates your fear of death. We've heard a lot about the threat of death since the borders closed and it became a real thing that locked us down (in this room, in our home, in this street, in this city) inside this

190

country. People on the news telling us Covid needed to be kept outside these islands because if it wasn't, many people would die. And far from us, there were deaths.

Your mother. Dear friends.

And everything changed, as Covid inevitably arrived on these islands anyway.

In the UK our relatives are no longer afraid of dying, though many people still are, and it has spread everywhere.

I arrived in this country to be with you, saturated in death.

And still you loved, love, will love me, even as more death arrives and surrounds us.

But on this morning you are not here.

Too many people you love have recently died.

Your mother. Dear friends.

We haven't been able to travel across the world to their funerals.

Your sister is gravely ill.

But it is still not possible to travel.

You need this blank moment, this not being-here.

But I am here to love you. I want to help you. To look after you.

I touch your arm. 'Baby?'

Your eyelids remain closed.

Thanatosis.

Lying on my side I take your hand. Your face is peaceful, as if inside you, there is a view of a lake, a mountain. A landscape of ferns. An open sky. Or perhaps you've gone somewhere far emptier, cleaner, clearer. I imagine you into a bleached-out landscape that's always light because the moon is brighter than we've ever known it to be. A landscape made entirely of salt, or snow, or chalk. A transparent boat with bedsheets for sails.

I whisper, 'Come back whenever you're ready to.'

A set of your watercolour paintings are pinned on the wall at the foot of our bed. These ones are images of the views from windows we have looked through together. The stormy coast at Dhuloch. The silver water at Queenstown. The Atlantic Ocean of Long Island—a place of bone fish. The wrought-iron fence in Glasgow. I imagine other scenes from other windows we've shared, the ones you didn't paint. The blue tarpaulin along our fence in Berhampore. The rooftops in York. The snowstorm outside your brother's flat in New

York. Your mother's garden. The high-rise windows full of closed-door-open-curtain hotel encounters in Chicago.

You are full of grief. You are tired of funerals being a set of pixelated figures dressed in black on a computer screen. The insubstantial weight of two-dimensional coffins. Flowers with no scent. Flattened music, so carefully chosen. Sequential photographs—baby to child to teenager to adult—blurring, glitching.

If we could talk, I'd want to talk about how it looks like the apocalypse everyone's always feared has already arrived and we should probably make a decision quite soon about who we want to be beside. Recently it seems that a lot of people can feel it; how we talk is changing. I often walk the streets of Wellington feeling contented in my invisibility because it means I can watch and overhear people. Many people have recently started to use catastrophic words in otherwise ordinary conversations. Apocalypse and which aisle to find soy sauce in at the supermarket. In the library, cookery books and Plague. Along the pavements, Climate Crisis and today's rain. Over the garden fence, Famine and the neighbours' new baby. And I can feel War in the distance late at night, like the buzz of too-loud too-bright electricity.

This conversation will have to wait a little longer. I think there's enough time as long as I pay attention to how the ground's feeling. I can tell when there's something significant below the surface of pavements, like running water, or people, or large hollow pipes. It vibrates through the soles of my feet, spreading upwards. I knew a couple of hours before the 7.8 earthquake that something frightening was about to happen. My body was full of adrenaline and an instinct for us to get outside and climb the nearest hill, chasing height and open skies. Hopefully I'll know when we need to run or fly away, before it's too late.

There's a stain of shadow around your eyes as if dreaming has made you tired. Emotions have got to come out of us somehow or they'll spread further inside as an overgrown tangle. No one can ever rescue anyone else by hacking their way through an internal tangle; it needs to be gently unteased.

Tangles take time and solitude. Grief needs air all around it.

Before tears can escape I close my eyes and follow you into darkness, keeping my distance just a little.

Beauty, Sleeping

I dream of being old and alone. I dream I am inside a fairy tale
that's gone wrong:

An old woman hides in her bed believing it is the only safe place
left in the world. She's overweight, so can last for a long time without
going to her kitchen for food. Outside her open window, the sky is
dark and there are the sounds of helicopters. Someone is screaming.
Perhaps everyone is screaming.

She covers her ears with a bunched-pillow, imagining her bed is
inside a fortress, a castle, a lonely boat. Everything has gone wrong
with the world. It happened fast, after happening slowly. People
thought there would be more time, but people were wrong. One
madman lost control while in charge of a country and made friends
with another country's madman who had also lost control. Now all
the madmen have lost control and become enemies with each other.
All of these madmen love only two things; power and death.

So now death is everywhere.

The few people who are still alive are locked in their homes, hiding
from viruses that travel via air. Water rises, burying stone and earth.
Air chokes with fumes, fighting with fire. Even from the safety of an
imagined fortress, or a castle, a lonely boat, or a bed, it is impossible
to ignore the smells of gas, pine trees, flesh and roses burning.

Loosening her grip on the pillow, the old woman hears the sound
of a man breathing in the gap between her bed and the wall. Death
must now feel this close, for everyone. She longs for something
powerful that isn't death. But the man rears up and she glimpses a
pale hooded face which is covered in scratches.

He has the word *prince* tattooed on his throat.

Regretting the fact that her knives are in the kitchen drawer, she
closes her eyes and pretends to already be dead.

Without asking permission, he kisses her and his lips taste of ash.

Biting his mouth, she enters a dream state, dragging him into it
with her.

She dreams of being in a crowded bar as she watches him getting his scratched hand stamped by the doorman.

He leaves his long coat in the cloakroom.

She stares at his thin thigh bones as he approaches the bar. She buys him a crimson-coloured cocktail, spikes it and smiles at him sweetly as he drinks.

When he's unstable on his feet, she kisses him and places a surgical mask over his face. He backs away from her and cowers in the corner, hollow eyes filled with mistrust.

And now she can forget him because he is nothing she wants.

She dreams of one hundred winters in a derelict city. In windowless supermarkets she eats tinned vegetables.

She empties seed packets into the gaps between crumbling paving stones, digs water out of broken drainpipes and climbs skeleton skyscrapers, rescuing earth from office plant pots, pouring it into bleached roof-gardens.

She dreams of one hundred springs. From the top of a church spire she whistles into the empty sky, calling for the birds, the insects, even the flies, to return.

She dreams of licking condensation from basement walls for one hundred summers.

She dreams of one hundred autumns and gathers knitted blankets from a block of apartments to make a shelter.

Sewing the blankets together with the unravelled threads of school shirts, she dreams of repair. She dreams of tree roots. She dreams of age.

She pricks her finger on a rusty needle.

The smell of her own infected blood wakes her. She wakes in her bedroom, as skinny as a witch.

There's a scythe lying on the floor, between the bed and the wall. She leans on it to lift her aching body from the bed.

Outside the open window, monstrous thorn bushes block the light with a mesh of thick leaves and rosebuds.

There is the sound of one bird cheeping, seeking a mate, or food, or a fight.

2021
After-Humans

Moon rising shining
Sun strikes a shaft of light.

Now reviving from Ground
a high-piping Nightingale cries, quench-Fire.

Time to flutter—
Leaves fall one by one.
A thousand Roses leave,
what have we to do with bluster?

Thistledown light,
I kiss your Ghost and you kiss mine.

As Ashes,
we land in this overgrown place.

Pale, wilderness, strange.

Disappear

Disappearing is easy. You just have to decide when to do it. The people all around you all think they can see who and what you are. But you've surrounded yourself with nothing of importance. You're with the wrong companion, perhaps. Or the wrong colleagues, the wrong friends, the wrong acquaintances. You're in the wrong house. The wrong job. You occupy a small space alongside all your wrong possessions, your wrong pet, wrong table, you sleep in the wrong half of the wrong bed. Anything can become a trap. The wrong home. The wrong lock for the wrong key.

If the things you once thought were important *all* now feel wrong, you are living in an invisible cage. It doesn't even matter how you got there, or whose fault it is.

The only way out is to disappear.

Invisible

My mum's recently told me that as a child I was too sensitive and she and my grandparents had no idea how I'd survive as an adult. My mum rarely cries. She can make tears disappear inside herself. She takes a deep breath and swallows them all in. She shows me how she does this when we talk on Skype, demonstrating the gulp, lips pressed tight, holding her breath.

I was a child who visibly cried. It was uncontrollable when I did. Did I feel more, or less, than the rest of my family? My three brothers must have learned how to not cry in front of other people. Did they attend private boy-lessons? How old were they, when they learned how to make tears vanish? My dad's moist green eyes only cried during the last few weeks of his life. It could have been real emotion, or the morphine and steroids. Either way, that's when he let us see his tears. Whether or not I was the only weeper in my family, as an adult I still cry uncontrollably, but as privately as a boy.

Disappear

What if all of the things you've been told are wrong with you, aren't really wrong at all?

You're too sensitive, too arrogant, too odd, too poor, too rich, too aggressive, too kind, too passive, too friendly, too clever, too silent, too talkative, too plain, too beautiful, too bright, too dull, too strange, too imaginative, too single-minded, too self-centred, too open, too closed, too addictive, too thick, too funny, too elegant, too clumsy, too pale, too filthy, too sexy, too angry, too soft, too emotional, too boring, too intellectual, too stupid, too much or too little…

If you decide to disregard all the things which are wrong with you, you'll realise you can walk away from any situation you've become trapped in. You might be drawn to solitary places, so you can work out what's right with you.

Islands. Long coastlines. Wildernesses.

Invisible

How to become invisible; be alone.

Think of a statue.

Think the statue into your whole body. All the way from slow stone heart to cold thumb-and-toe-edges.

Become still and become closed.

Shut your eyes, because statues are blind. Stop listening. Shut your mouth to hunger.

Let stone creep through the body's tissues, blood, bones.

Don't move until someone shouts sound into your stone ears.

Disappear

How to disappear; choose the right moment to leave.

Be alert to signs—the rightness of this moment could show up anywhere. A sliver of sunlight after days of rain. The call of a migrating bird, revealing the direction.

It will be something small, something meaningful for you alone.

A miniature snail you avoid stepping on.

A moth you rescue from having a dry death indoors.

The strange shape of a rogue cloud.

Invisible

It's 2009. I've been diagnosed with PTSD. When I don't eat enough, I get so dizzy that the edges of all things blur with light. I float in pure electricity. There's always danger when there's too much electricity. If I do this for long enough, I'll frazzle like the element inside a lightbulb. I have to fix this one myself. Find the on and off switch, for hunger. No one can look directly at me when I'm this light and burning and breakable.

I want to disappear. It would be so easy to do it this way. I wasn't always this fragile. Something invisible is very slowly breaking me. I see it and can't see it. Z says she loves me.

It's 2012. I'm slowly and carefully withdrawing from all my medication and not telling anyone. Not my doctor. Not Z. I need to know if I can survive without these triplets: Dosulepin. Zopiclone. Valium.

It's 2013. I'm leaving in search of an open sky. Daylight.

Disappear

Save any money you earn—you need to use it to buy time instead of possessions.

Return any possessions you've borrowed from friends and acquaintances. Do this quietly, without fuss. If they ask questions, smile, make eye contact, but avoid answering. Remember that most people prefer to talk about themselves over and above any other subject. So, ask them questions and listen to their answers.

No one remembers you, unless you *make* them remember you.

You can decide not to.

Invisible

It's the mid-1990s. A hotel room in Hampshire. The room is full of cousins, aunts and uncles, parents and brothers and grandparents—they're having an anniversary. It's the night of a celebration meal, most of us have only just arrived. There's a small clock on a bedside cabinet. It's four-thirty.

I'm perched on a cousin's single bed in the middle of this hotel room. I'm still wearing my coat and scarf. There are far too many beds and smells. Bags and damp coats and granny's poshest perfume and one uncle's aftershave and another's egg sandwich and a rose candle smell and all of these smells make this green-red bedspread feel scratchy. There's the white sound of a toilet flushing and the pink sound of my mum talking and my auntie laughing and my granny singing and my brother murmuring something to my dad with an orange sound and my littlest cousin's tickling the two middle cousins and the sound is sharp bursts of pale blue and there's a telephone ringing somewhere—is a window open, no. Just a crack. There's a brown aeroplane sound and a purple bus sound and a lilac guitar sound and the carpet is green and purple tartan and where is the guitar sound coming from when there aren't any instruments and everyone is speaking and laughing in colour. My dark-haired cousin A and his carer aren't here yet. I haven't seen A for years. He doesn't speak or make much eye contact. He could rollerblade from the very first time he put skates on. Never even fell. He must be a balancing genius. I swipe my fingertips across the scratchy bedspread as if I could turn its texture into paint and then I'd not notice anything else in this room apart from the picture I was painting. There's no air moving. The clock still says four-thirty. Is the battery dead?

My mum's voice speaks close to my ear, 'You're very quiet.'

I reappear.

A is here, forehead-to-forehead with Granny. She's beaming to see him. He's good at eye-contact with her, because she's familiar.

I wish I lived nearer to him.

The clock says five-thirty.

I don't know where I've been for the last hour.

Disappear

Get rid of your remaining possessions. Pack only what you need for survival and one small thing for comfort.

Release yourself from object-nostalgia—instead, conjure memories. If you can't remember something vividly, it isn't worth remembering. Anything you once loved can be found in memory fragments, like a trick of the light. A colour. A familiar tune or picture.

It is best to have a plan for at least the first night after leaving—somewhere safe to sleep. Make sure there's water and food. A door with a lock, a key in your hand.

Invisible

What is the difference between having no empathy and having too much empathy?

As a child I had to be told I could only say someone had 'said' something, if they'd 'said' it out loud. Knowing what someone thinks or feels isn't enough. Even when it's obvious.

Thoughts have to remain invisible till they are spoken.

Why?

Disappear

If, when disappearing, you need to say goodbye to someone, set a time limit for this conversation. Let them talk first and without interruption. Repeat the most moving thing they have said and speak it kindly to them so they know you have listened. If you need to disappear it's not their fault. It's not your fault either, but it is best to try to avoid conversations about blame. When you disappear, remember it is polite to softly close the door behind you.

Invisible

My dad was a teacher at the local primary school. He taught my brothers and me aged seven to nine as we passed through his class. Sometimes I wouldn't take the yellow bus home, but would wait for a lift home with him when he'd finished for the day. This was often late. My friend B lived with her nana, who was the school cleaner. B's nana had got her piano lessons but they lived in a flat with no piano. While I was waiting for my dad, B would practice on the school piano.

The upright piano was in a large room used for school dinners, school tellings-off, school gym, cubs and brownies and the annual Christmas party. After school, B's nana would slide a heavy machine back, forth, back, shining up the whole floor with a deep hovercraft hum. B would sit at the piano with her back to the room, playing from a book of sheet music. And behind their backs, on the dull patches of floor which hadn't yet been polished, I'd be dancing to B's music. She was playing notes, but I could hear words inside them. A tune called 'Sleeping Cat' was my favourite. Once I knew the title, each note became a word and I would dance unseen to the words. The sound of a piano playing the word 'sleeping' moves both wrists and one ankle. The sound of a piano playing the word 'cat' moves the neck and the fingertips. Dancing unseen to the words hidden in the notes of piano music along with the rhythmic sounds of a floor-polisher was as close to flying as I could get, my whole body feeling sounds and words, breath-less and breath-more.

One day when I was dancing, B's nana must have looked over her shoulder and noticed me. She spoke to my dad as he left his classroom.

'She's really graceful. She should be going to dance lessons.'

He laughed and said, 'I wish she was graceful at home.'

I cried in the car because I hadn't known I was clumsy. What else hadn't he told me? I felt hyper-visible to other people and hyper-invisible to myself.

B's nana didn't give up. She gave my dad a phone number for a dance class. He and my mum asked me about dancing. Red-faced, I said I wanted to learn. They didn't think it was a good idea, but they didn't say so out loud. My brothers teased me about being a prissy girl. I bit my lip and kept thinking about music and words and flying.

The Dance Class was in the nearest town, Stranraer. It was inside a low-ceilinged room with no windows. There was a row of girls wearing up-hair, matching leotards and pumps. I was barefoot and my tangled hair was down. There was no piano, or polishing machine. There was no shiny and dull floor, there was no B or her nana with their backs turned.

There were Positions and we were put into Groups. I was the tallest in the tall group. We were told we had to be Jack Frost in Second Position and we had to, 'Kick the Legs without Bending the Knees'. The cassette machine played the sounds of tin violins and can flutes. The tune was a piece of classical music about winter, but the music wasn't right for the words Jack or Frost.

The word Jack was moving elbows.

Frost was a clench in the jaw and left knee. The tin can sounds from the cassette player were a curved movement, the body curled in on itself.

I stood up straight, kicked my legs and tried not to hear the music. I thought about Jack Frost and how cold he must feel. Crisp and shining and icy. Like snow. Like clean teeth.

The teacher was frowning so I smiled icicles at her dancing pumps. My face was burning because the borrowed leotard I was wearing was too small. They could all see far too much of my bum. I tried to pull it down but the pinching elastic rose up again.

The other girls in the tall group whispered to each other as I smiled winter at them.

They didn't smile back.

I left quickly so I could be invisible again.

My brothers stopped doing impressions of clumsy ballerinas after about five days.

Disappear

Once you have disappeared, switch off all your electronic devices.

After three weeks, no one you know will call your cell phone.

After eight weeks, no one you know will text you.

After three months, no one you know will email you more than once a year.

When you think it is safe to turn on your electronic devices because no one will be communicating with you, you can use them to research new places to live.

House-sits. Holiday lets in winter. Caravans. Spare rooms. Tents. Deserted buildings.

Invisible

McMillenstink was a name given to a whole-playground game, a slur against a desperately poor family. Someone touched one of the McMillen siblings to catch their stink and passed it around shouting 'McMillenstink'. It was played like tig or tag, all the kids spreading the smell of this family from one to the next, a virus.

I wouldn't play this game. It made me cry each night, thinking about it.

Instead, I shared any lolly I could get hold of with the pale McMillen sisters and made sure everyone in the playground saw me do it.

A thin paper stick in a square block of red sugar.

Red sugar was love. Red sugar was anger.

Red sugar was passed from my filthy mouth

to C McMillen's filthy mouth

to D McMillen's filthy mouth
to E McMillen's filthy mouth
to my filthy mouth...
until it was sucked right down to
nothing.

Disappear

After you have disappeared, the people who once knew you are still surrounded by all the other people they've always been distracted by.

You'll think about them far more often than they think about you.

This might make you sad, sometimes.

Drop a tear in an empty glass jar.

If you ever cry enough to fill the whole jar with tears, hold it up and look at the sky.

The clouds look the same as always.

The birds are distorted because they disappear, reappear, disappear, reappear around the curve of the glass.

You can miss them too
but only for a moment.

Invisible

I don't know what it is I can't see. But there's something there, just out of sight. It hisses into my ears like electricity. It's getting louder, closer than ever before.

Disappear

How to disappear; stop wanting anything from anyone else.

Invisible

When you're invisible, no one thinks about you. If no one is thinking of you, no one can tell you anything true or false. No one can blame you. No one can love you. No one can hurt you. No one can tell you who you are. If you've managed to disappear *and* become invisible, you can make yourself up.

If you're invisible because you're a ghost, you'll be everywhere and nowhere all at the same time. You'll be far too busy with things living people know nothing about, to bother with visibility. This is probably what's happened to my dad.

If, however, you are an extrovert who misses being visible, you can bandage yourself and reappear whenever you want to. But no one will believe in you. If you wear a sheet, no one will believe in you either. Why do ghosts and invisible people only wear pale things?

Whether you are an invisible ghost, or an invisible living person, if it's important to you that people can see you, you might consider wearing something colourful.

Flamingo wings.

Kingfisher feathers.

A toucan beak.

Invisible

I learned how to draw so that invisible things became visible. When I was a child, I drew other children's faces. Once I'd drawn them, they'd always smile at me, because they'd remember that I'd seen them. I drew some things because I wanted there to be more of them in the world. Cats, trees, the ocean, clouds, rain, seahorses, shells. I drew spiders to train myself not to be scared of them. As teenager I drew bottles of poison, snakes, tangled branches, skulls. As I got older I drew witches, helicopters, broomsticks, hot air balloons, dragonflies, aeroplanes. I drew women who could see the shapes of air moving around them.

Recently, I've been drawing birds flying in swirling lines—gradients, ocean currents.

Flocks of graphite birds, swerving into flight. Beckoning ghosts to join them.

Flocks of ghosts—drawn in visible and invisible ink.

Disappear

When you've disappeared, as long as you are protected from weather and have enough food to keep you alive, you can do whatever you want. All of the time.

After a while, you might become lonely. And after a while of being lonely you'll understand what love really is. Your eyes will be wide open and you'll feel love constantly for all kinds of creatures— not just human creatures, but bird creatures, plant and stone and animal creatures, elemental creatures which are just out of sight in the wind and running waters, in fires and in the soil...If you don't resist this feeling, soon you'll feel like you're entirely made of love. You will disappear into it. It will be beautiful.

Invisible

Unless you want to be followed, do not steal anything from anyone else.

If you *do* want to be followed, steal something from the person you want to be followed by. You will stop being invisible, but only to them. Send them ransom notes and photos of the thing you've stolen, from different locations.

You will steal their heart.

Let them steal something that belongs to you. Turn around, and follow them.

Let them steal your heart.

If the one you fall in love with can see you whether you're invisible or not, you'll have finally found the right companion.

Disappear

I'm having an autism spectrum assessment because there are so many things I don't understand, mainly about loneliness. It takes a long time to be tested. I'm scared about what any answer or non-answer will mean. I'm scared that this kind of knowledge will be so overwhelming I will vanish. I might not go through with it.

Visibility

What would it be like to become visible again, after disappearing from one kind of life and finding another? For a long time after leaving Z I couldn't think about the past or the future. Now, some memories are returning. I don't seem to be able to lie. I have become quieter and have stopped pretending it's easy to talk to new people. Many people don't see me because I'm good at being partially, if not completely, invisible. But if I was to let myself become visible, you might see something like this—

In most group situations I either pretend not to be terrified, or am tongue-bound, or want to cry because too often I feel strange or odd. I twirl my hair all the time and can't stop it. If I have a role and something useful to say, I'll speak clearly so I don't have to talk for too long. In most group situations, I say nothing at all.

When I can, I'll ask questions instead of answering them. Sometimes I don't talk for ages. If I'm talking about a subject I love, I'm confident, but I only love two subjects. Can't do sums. Don't know how to make new friends. I love writing and art and my doctorate earned me a place on the Dean's List. I've published three novels, inventing new worlds in each of them.

I will never be unfaithful to Morgan. She can see me even when I'm invisible. When we first got together she kidnapped my sunglasses and I stole her favourite t-shirt. We exchanged ransom notes and got married. Morgan wore blue gloves and a suit. I wore a scarlet dress and red shoes and we were both visible for our whole wedding day.

I could be the kindest person you'll ever meet. Having too much empathy, I avoid being around groups of people for too long. I need to hide afterwards, often in a completely dark room. I think very deeply, often looping my thoughts to re-play the conversations, about every person who speaks to me. I won't deliberately hurt anyone. I still think in magical ways like a child. It's probably quite hard to get to know me unless you're a cat. I'm often sad about this, because I've felt lonely my whole life.

My favourite words to use when I'm writing stories are *pale*, *wilderness* and *strange* because each of these words can disappear and reappear. They belong in fairy tales. Each has a different musical sound and movement in the body.

Pale has the sound of an oboe reed and a slight tilt of the head.

Wilderness is a tangle of blocky percussion and a ripple through the shoulders.

Strange has the sound of a bowed saw and is the ball of the foot, running away.

Thirteen Words for Loneliness

Despane– The loneliness of feeling misunderstood, unloved or unheard by someone who used to understand, love or listen.

Starn– Craving something or someone to be there but knowing it's/ they're not. Wanting to bite something.

Youache– Where a specific person is missed and only their physical presence will cure the ache of missing them.

Ignornly– The kind of loneliness that other people notice, but don't mention to the person they think is lonely. Their expression shows sympathy, but also a little wariness, as if loneliness could be contagious.

Solilone– A type of melancholia experienced while gazing at a wide-skied landscape. A longing for strangeness, for the unreal or the surreal to appear.

Idealone– A hankering for an imagined scenario—where it's the idea of the situation that causes the loneliness. For example, the 'ideal' of the perfect friend sitting opposite on the sofa, laughing over wine and confessions and saying all of the right things.

Achiposs– The ache of missing out on experiencing something beautiful, because it is impossible.

Disampty– Where the immediate environment is problematic – usually in practical ways. The rubbish split all over the floor, the smoke alarm is going off, work is waiting, the clock is ticking, the umbrella's broken, it's lashing with rain and there's no one else around.

Crowdsad– Felt while around many other people. Crying while walking along streets crammed with strangers, feeling unable to speak during a burbling conversation in which others are talking loudly and not leaving any gaps.

Feartrap– when alone, overactive fears producing images of other people becoming monstrous.

Priclash– Keeping emotions or secrets private while desperately wanting to let them out.

Xiley– The loneliness of ears: usually during unexpected silence. For example, when any music player suddenly ceases to work and refuses to be fixed.

Lonmyth– the belief that no one cares / is interested, without any effort to allow people to care or show that they're interested.

Ghosts are Repetitions

When there are no human mouths left to speak stories,

no one will care
                    or pretend to care

    I'll hold ice-cubes in my palm
    while wondering if ghosts speak in a language
    of echoes, rhythms, repetitions?

it will be raining and raining and raining
and there will be no boats to take us to dry land
we will be huddled under tin roofs
and old songs will be sung on the wind
in languages we must never forget were stolen

the childhood stories we remember
will be retold by lost and flying things
by ghosts, or birds

(these flighty things, like stories, will always travel)

as echoes,
   rhythms,

      repetitions.

Tales of Birds and Ghosts

Three Short Journeys through Storytelling Theories written by Ghosts.

There are only Two Stories

The ghost, Leo Tolstoy, famously said,

'All great literature is one of two stories; a man goes on a journey or a stranger comes to town.'

A man goes on a journey a stranger comes to town a man stays where he is a stranger leaves town a dead man goes on a journey a ghost comes to town a journey leaves a man a town welcomes a stranger a ghost man ends a journey a town evicts a stranger a woman goes on a journey a bird comes to town a woman journeys with a bird a town welcomes a ghost a dead woman ends a journey a stranger bird leaves town a ghost woman comes to town a bird goes on a journey a bird comes to town a ghost goes on a journey a ghost leaves a town of strangers a journey leaves a bird a dead town becomes a ghost a stranger journeys with a bird a ghost becomes a stranger a bird goes on a journey to town a ghost journeys with a bird a stranger comes to a ghost town a ghost stays where it is a bird goes to a stranger town a ghost journeys with a bird a town goes on a journey a ghost leaves a journey a woman traps a bird a man comes to town a ghost catches a man a bird woman journeys with a ghost a town is full of strangers

a ghost is a journeying bird.

The Seven Plots

The ghost, Christopher Booker, wrote the book *The Seven Basic Plots*. (2004) Every story in the world is supposed to fit to one of these plots. It took Booker thirty-four years to research and write this book. He must have been confident there were only seven.

Overcoming the Monster

The bird doesn't know what the monster looks or smells like.
The monster has a metal-zing-chemical-zang-scent. It is half-liquid and half-colour.
It has stolen the rainbows right out of the sky.
The bird is caught by the monster.
The monster glues the bird's feathers together and creeps inside its body.
The bird becomes a ghost and flies away.

Tragedy

In the human body, white blood cells are the last things to die.
They are supposed to help fight infection.

The Quest

There is white netting suspended in the sky. It is often mistaken for clouds.
This netting is made of multiple ghosts that have been created simultaneously. They have rushed into the sky with no sense of direction and thinned into threads.
Any ghost or bird who chooses to become a rescuer of waifs might accept the quest; to untangle the net and set the ghosts free.
But the ghosts *are* the net. They are thread-thin. Transparent.
When exhausted, they fall as rain.

Rags to Riches

Birds tear rags into threads and weave them through twigs and leaves to build their nests. They warm the nest with feathers and lay eggs.
Egg anatomy; an eggshell surround. Inside: thin and thick albumen, yolk, chalaza and airspace.
A blastodisc splits and splits and splits inside a golden yolk.
Growing and growing and growing a new bird.

Rebirth

The heart starts to beat before blood begins to form.

Beating death beating death beating death tubes death folded death set death heart death formed death heart death chambers death four death weeks nine death chambers death heart death lower death two death ventricles death forms death tube death top death chambers death two death upper death, atria death forms death back death towards death up death folds death tube death bottom death death bend death twist death tubes death weeks death over death beat to death begin death flow death to death begin death blood death together death fuse death tubes death embryo death in death grown death heart death form death tubes death two death pregnancy death weeks death five death

birth five birth weeks birth pregnancy birth two birth tubes birth form birth heart birth grown birth in birth embryo birth tubes birth fuse birth together birth blood birth begin birth to birth flow birth begin birth to birth beat birth over birth weeks birth tubes birth twist birth bend birth bottom birth tube birth folds birth up birth towards birth back birth forms birth atria birth upper birth two birth chambers birth top birth tube birth forms birth ventricles birth two birth lower birth heart birth chambers birth nine birth weeks birth four birth chambers birth heart birth formed birth heart birth set birth folded birth tubes birth beating birth beating birth beating.

The heart starts to beat before blood begins to form.

Comedy

If all human hearts became birds, they would become lost in storms and would peck and scratch while searching for the right bird. Every day, another storm. Every night, another wrong bird.

Peck here, scratch there, the right one is out there somewhere, high in the gales.

One night they might hear the sound of snoring and tell themselves they've heard a sweet-heartbeating ditty they could sip nectar and dance along to. *Almost* right is right enough.

And they would find the wrong bird snoring a song they didn't feel and name it the right bird because they hoped for their search to be over. They wanted to look like the kinds of lovebirds all the other storm-crossed birds could aspire to. Ignore the droppings and dirty feather lining, their nest appears perfectly woven from the outside.

The perfect nest is what they see, so that is what they have. And they laugh and they laugh and they laugh so much that they appear to be *almost* laughing.

Voyage and Return

Entanglement occurs when particles are created at the same moment and place. (birth/death)

Ghosts might never have heard about entangled particles becoming separated and yet being still connected, or any version of 'spooky action at a distance,'[7] but that's exactly what is going on. Separation and entanglement are instinctive states of being, for ghosts.

This is how it works; a ghost splits into several parts. It divides itself across multiple times and places. One part of this ghost kicks and stamps around the house it was born in, another part simultaneously

---

7 Albert Einstein. Another ghost.

kicks and stamps and twirls in the room the ghost last occupied when it was living. Another part of the ghost twirls as it climbs a mountain to hum at the moon, another climbs to the surface of a lake and sings at the rain. Another part air-kisses a black and white photograph of its spouse, another tries and fails to pick a rose with its transparent lips. One part of the ghost crawls through the most ancient of caves, examining the recent drawings on rock. Another part crawls around a future-room filled with an artificial light so intense it makes all invisible things, visible.

Ghosts occupy multiple times and places, all of which contain some kind of density or intensity. Pitch, tone, colour, temperature, emotions, darkness, light.

Ghosts voyage and return, return and voyage, voyage and return.

Rules of Three (Transformation Tales)

To explore 'rules of three' see the works of the ghost: Vladimir Propp, *The Morphology of the Folk Tale*.

Albert Einstein, the ghost mentioned previously (who wrote about 'spooky action at a distance') is also reported to have said: 'If you want your child to be intelligent, read them fairy stories. If you want your child to be more intelligent, read them more fairy stories.'

If you want your ghosts to be intelligent, read them spooky stories about distant birds.

Accumulation: Three events

A ragged bird goes to a golden cage and asks to be let in.
It is told by the cage that it is not wearing appropriate attire.
A ragged bird goes to a golden cage and demands to be let in.
It is told by the cage that if could hire some peacock feathers, it should come back tomorrow.
A ragged bird goes to a golden cage and burns like a phoenix.
The cage melts down and down and down until it becomes a golden nest.
The phoenix steps in and lays a burning egg.
The egg hatches three fat pigeons who believe they deserve gold.

Contrasting: straw, twig, brick

It is cold at night, in winter.
A thin ghost with no home asks if it can move into a straw house.
The three fat pigeons who live in the straw house don't want to help the ghost.
The ghost blows their straw house away.

It is cold at night, in winter.
A thin ghost with no home asks if it can move into a twig house.
The three fat pigeons who live in the twig house don't want to help the ghost.
The ghost blows their twig house away.
It is cold at night, in winter.
A thin ghost with no home asks if it can move into a brick house.
The three fat pigeons who live in the brick house look out of the windows at the ghost.
The ghost looks back.
And it blows and it blows and it blows itself out.

Final Three: wrong: opposite wrong: final right.

When the ghost has blown itself out, the three fat pigeons go outside and peck at the ground where the ghost was standing.
In the grass there's a white powdery substance they've never tasted before.
Is it poison, is it chemical, is it salt? They eat and eat and eat it because it is new and they want and want and want it.
Whatever the powder is, it tastes of winter.
The fat pigeons lose their appetite for new things and become thin.
They don't even want their house any more.
Too many strange noises on cold winter nights.
And since the ghost blew itself out, every night feels like winter.
The pigeons eat white sugar, trying to fatten themselves up again.
One pigeon says, 'Is gunpowder white? Is it? Does it taste of winter?'
The other two pigeons do not reply.
One night there is an earthquake. The brick house cracks right through the wall which holds up the chimney.
One pigeon flies to the north, where the winter is even colder and its heart turns to ice.
One pigeon flies to the south, where the ocean is too wide and drops from the sky into water.
The other pigeon dies of shock inside its broken house.

It dies white as gunpowder

white as a page with no story

white as a ghost with no home.

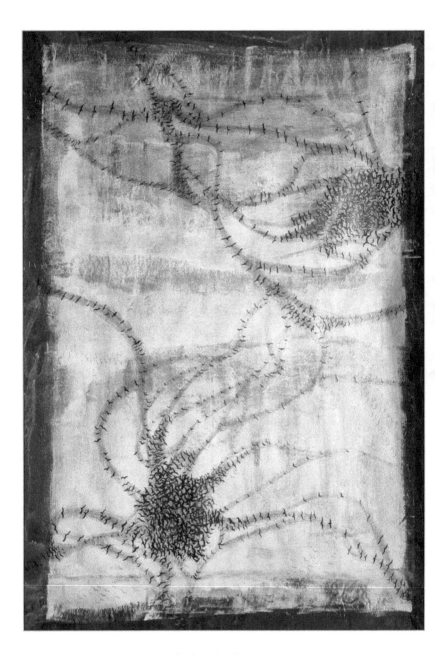

Flock of Ghosts VI

2021
Friday the 13th of August

This is only the time of writing.
The number of new ghosts is rising so fast.
There are 621,000 more ghosts than there should be, in the USA.
There is one more ghost than there should be, in Western Sahara.
There are 430,000 more ghosts than there should be, in India.

This is no time for writing about anything other than death.
I can sense the edges of the lone ghost in Western Sahara from here in New Zealand.
It floats above a rock in the desert.
It has no feet. It used to walk everywhere but now it can't find its way home.

In its transparent hands, it clutches 4.35 million pale threads.
The threads twist upwards into the sky and make a vast web across the whole world.
Each thread leads to another ghost who is one more ghost than there should be.
The ghost in Western Sahara floats above a rock in the desert, counting threads.

The sun crosses the sky.
The sun rises and falls again.
The moon crosses the sky.
The moon rises and falls again.

And all the while the ghost floats above a rock in the desert, clutching more and more threads.
It's waiting for a sign—some small vibration along a thread.
It's hunting for proof it's not alone.

Ghosts Have No Feet

I

There's a broken pair of shoes on the edge of Adelaide Road in Wellington, New Zealand. Block heels. Black elastic. Teenage girl shoes. A seventeen-eighteen year old? I don't know why I think that. The heels of both shoes are smashed, as if they've been run over by a car. They appeared on the same night that there was a fatal stabbing at a teenage party in Christchurch. I look for blood on the road but don't see any.

II

As a young woman I lived in Carlisle in the UK. Three different student rooms in three different terraced houses over one year. I was only eighteen and loved the city so much I wanted to belong to it. One way of doing this was to allow myself to touch it physically, and to allow the city to touch me back. This meant feeling the pavement beneath my bare feet. Letting the texture of the pavement harden my soles. Occasionally releasing a spit or spot of blood, claimed by grit or glass. I walked around barefoot for months.

Strangers would walk right past me, looking downwards. Avoiding eye contact they'd say, 'No shoes.'

Just that. 'No shoes.' As if there was something deeply wrong. As if I was almost-visible.

III

2010. In Brighton, England, along all the walking-routes to secondary schools and all the walking-routes to pubs and clubs, shoes with the laces tied together hang from overhead electricity wires. All these school kids and big kids will have had to walk home without shoes. I worry about bullying and fun and how closely together these two things live.

IV

August 2021. The voices of social media and emails:

'The teenagers all have mental health problems now. Well, I suppose everyone does.'

'I'm so sorry I gave birth to my son in the end times.'

'The birds are much louder now. Especially the tūī. Since the tree fell in the storm. Since there's less traffic. Have you noticed?'

'I had to be resuscitated. I don't think I told you that.'

'There's no immunity if someone is immunocompromised. Even with vaccines.'

'You'll be over next year though, won't you?'

'We can all move around freely now.'

'Elimination is impossible. We just have to live with it. So will you.'

'Why aren't you all vaccinated yet? I thought New Zealand was good at this.'

'Nothing is important any more. But we're still remembering stupid memories. Well, any memories at all, from before. But there's also this urgent feeling that if we don't remember them all now, soon we won't have any memories at all.'

'I am so *over* hearing people grumbling about not seeing their families for a couple of months. It's been over two years for me now. Longer for you.'

'Everyone in New Zealand must be so smug. With Covid and Jacinda and everything. I suppose there's a Jacinda in every country. Many Jacindas. But people have to vote for her.'

'I miss you.'

'The apocalypse hasn't started recently. It started many years ago.'

'Covid's come back to New Zealand. Inevitable, really.'

'When are you moving back home to the UK?'

'We're not doing too well, are we? Humans.'

'We have no idea, here in New Zealand, what the rest of the world is going through.'

'We just want to spend time with family this year, not make new friends.'

V

When I was a child my family lived in a rural area in Scotland around six miles from the nearest villages of Leswalt in one direction and Kirkcolm in the other. We lived eight miles beyond an end-of-the-line town called Stranraer. We four siblings each had two pairs of shoes—one for school and everyday use, the other a pair of sandshoes for school gym. When I was about ten years old I got wellies for the first time. They were the brightest red. I wore them with my party dress. I wore them with dungarees. I wore them with pyjamas and with a swimming costume. I wore them in puddles, in nettles, in the woods, in the Irish Sea, on jagged rocks, on grass-cracked roads, in wheat fields, in the ruins of old cottages, in tangled brambles on verges.

VI

There's a pair of work boots on the pavement beside a lamp-post in Berhampore, Wellington. Toes worn. Scuffed. Shoelaces tied into double bows. Damp from three days and nights of rain. They are arranged with such precision that no one has tried to move them, not even the wind. The worker must have placed them there after work one night and climbed the lamp-post. Then, they opened their hidden wings and flew upwards, beyond the lightbulb.

VII

When I walk around Wellington with Morgan she often laughs in response to my pointing out empty shoes on urban pavements, wires, fences, walls, roads.

She tells me, 'It's strange you notice shoes everywhere.'

I reply, 'It's far stranger that there *are* shoes everywhere.'

She says, 'But I never see them unless I'm with you.'

VIII

I remember binding my mother's feet when she was my daughter. I broke them at the arch, folded the toes under each foot, trying to halve the feet in length. I bandaged her folded feet tightly in wet fabric. Exactly the way it had to be done, or I would ruin all her chances in life.

There is no reason for this memory. My mother has never been my daughter. Both she and I were born in the UK within the past eighty years, not China in the past.

Her feet aren't broken. They are one size smaller than mine. I have often bought her new slippers or the softest socks for her birthdays.

When I was in my late-twenties I studied reflexology at night school. When I needed to do case studies for the course, I went north to visit my mum and dad in their home in Scotland and gave them foot massages.

Now it is 2021. My dad is a ghost. He's gone somewhere I can't find him. I haven't seen my mum for over three years. But I can still remember the frail texture of the soles of their feet.

IX

When I was around nine, I used to have a reoccurring dream about walking along the pavements of the nearest town with my family. The pavement cut my bare feet, and in this dream I could feel excruciating pain. My shoes had fallen off somewhere but I'd not noticed. I'd cry out to my family to wait for me, but they never heard my voice. Their long silhouettes walked away through grey streets into brightness. The dilemma was always whether to go back and find my shoes, knowing I'd lose my family, or to follow them with bleeding feet. I always went back for the shoes. When I'd managed to find at least one shoe, I would spend the rest of the dream hopping through the grey town filled with shadows, looking for my lost family.

X

Up until Summer 2013 I lived in Brighton with my wife Z, who loved a particular brand of shoes. They were the kinds of high-heeled shoes that might belong to an extrovert princess—all glitter and kitsch kittens and pin-up girls and pin-stripes and polka-dots and pearls. The kind of shoes that would be dropped on grand stairways on the way out of parties, to encourage pursuit.

Over the fifteen years we were together, for many birthdays, Christmases and anniversaries, I bought Z a pair of these shoes. She wore a pair of them on our wedding day— Friday the 13th of October, a date I chose for fun or thoughtless irony because it was unlucky. Z bought this brand of shoes for herself as well, on e-Bay, in the summer sales, in the winter sales.

We lived in a small rented flat, and by the time I left Z owned around fifty pairs. They were stacked in their shoeboxes in the bedroom, beneath our shared clothing rail, and worn only on special occasions. As Z became louder over the years I became quieter. When I eventually disappeared, I donated my possessions to charity shops.

I sometimes still imagine the gap on the clothing rail left by my absent clothing.

All those boxes of rarely-worn princess shoes, exposed.

Waiting to dance, waiting to be pursued by princes.

XI

I often walk around Wellington alone. At times I feel like a ghost because I don't belong here. I'm a hunting ghost. I hunt for the tiny lumps of grit between paving stones. I hunt for the holes in concrete. I hunt for underground pipes and wires and dropped scarves and broken chain jewellery. I hunt for empty shoes and imagine they belong to people who have flown away, upwards. I hunt for boarded-up doors. I hunt for derelict buildings and broken twigs that resemble wind-swept trees and I hunt for flax flower stems. I hunt for strands of long hair caught in wire fences and I hunt for the sound of a helicopter landing on the hospital roof. I hunt for cobwebs woven so randomly they can't possibly catch anything and I hunt for all the creatures which like me, shouldn't be here: chaffinches, rabbits, sparrows, cats, blackbirds, rats.

I listen for native birds: pīwakawaka, tūī, tauhou, ruru, and try to learn their songs. I talk to all the birds as I keep an eye out for all the things I've been subtly warned about, like stink bugs and black mould and patched gangs and tuneless bagpipes and racism and leaky homes and synthetic cannabis.

I hunt for the smallest cracks in walls, the ones no one else has noticed yet. Even after five years the sense of the ground shifting still frightens me. I wear boots, even in summer. But all of my boots feel as if the soles are too thin, too insubstantial. I try to walk as lightly as a ghost, so that when the earth quakes, I can leap instead of fall.

XII

The farm across the road from my childhood home was a dairy farm, and I'll never forget the wails of cows when their calves were taken away. Beef farmers also used to drive their cattle along the road beside our house. My family were vegetarians.

On winter mornings the cows' breath hung in the air.

When they walked at their own pace, their exhaled breath was a halo.

It became a phantom when they were forced to run.

XIII

My dad's empty jacket and gardening hat still hang on a hook in his empty study in Scotland.

Apart from a red silk shirt that I claimed, another hat I gave to his sister, and whatever my mum or brothers might have kept, that's the last of his clothing.

After he died in 2014 his clothes were packed up and given to charity shops, which is where most of them came from in the first place.

I keep thinking about his footwear.

His boots, shoes and slippers were bought new and would have been worn only by him.

Now strangers walk around in his shoes.

They limp slightly as their feet fail to adjust to the indentations of his soles.

To the shape of empty space.

XIV

Morgan loves New Zealand. Walking around Wellington with her hand in the crook of my arm, she helps me see it through her eyes.

Perhaps I won't always feel like a ghost here.

Seeing what she loves about this city is like seeing floodlights go on, illuminating, adding colour.

She lights up the sunlight on tin rooftops.

She colours the distant mountains indigo and ochre.

She shows me the lights of windows rising up dark hills, the outlines of shadow-trees.

At Island Bay after a storm we can't walk along the beach because it will sting our feet.

Instead, we crouch on concrete steps to look at translucent blue pieces of jellyfish scattered across grey sand.

XV

It's summer, 2018. At night-time at Duppa Street in Wellington, Morgan lights a fire in our garden. To stop the mozzies sucking our blood, we tuck our trousers into our boots.

We listen to the melancholic calls of the ruru, a small owl that belongs here.

Morgan looks up.

Above us there are stars. So many stars. More than I've ever seen.

The full moon is the centre point of a shimmering ring.

It's surrounded by a halo of its own exhaled breath.

The Ghost in the Room

Mask

Before I open my eyes each morning I mentally list all the things I've done wrong. This is so I don't think about them all day.

There are many things I need to list because before I have language, I can make the wrong things vanish.

I'm forty-nine and I still wake into thinking like a child.

After I wake in the morning and list the wrong things, I can forget them.

Mask

Before I open my eyes each morning I remember my dad is dead.

My dad so suddenly died that he still feels suddenly dead. We were told back then he would die within weeks or days. I kept saying months or weeks, and he and my mum and three brothers and the cancer nurses kept having to correct me. I'm the only daughter. Too emotional.

Perhaps every parent's death feels sudden, to their children.

There's a rip in the sky he's gone away through.

I'm half-pulled through, after him.

Morgan lies sleeping beside me. In this tiny white-walled bedroom, the brown blind lets in a sliver of pre-dawn light.

The softness of the sheet across my ankles, the first call of an unidentifiable bird.

The smooth skin of her shoulder.

These real things hide my dad from me.

These real things pull me back from the rip and hold me here.

Mask

When I wake in the morning I open my eyes and see something which isn't there. There's a ghost in the corner of the bedroom. She's blurring like a shadow against the white wall. She is half-lying, half-sitting up there on a high corner shelf that doesn't exist. She's been there before dawn for the past three days. She disappears as it gets light so she'll be gone soon. Those three other mornings, I've ignored her.

But today I'm curious.

I want to know why she's here *now*.

Mask

The ghost is wearing a grey nightgown and is curled across an invisible corner shelf, hugging her knees.

She looks like me at age fourteen—same nightgown, same awkward body.

Her brown hair is a tangled mask.

She hasn't quite got to the age I was when I started dying my hair or wearing makeup.

The ghost hides her naked face.

She has heard of the names of the face-drawing materials—foundation. Eye liner, lipstick, eyeshadow. Blusher, mascara, powder.

But she doesn't yet know *how* to draw a face over her own face.

How to know when the layers are thick enough.

Mask

—to protect others from our breath.

Before I open my eyes I remember the pandemic. We're in lockdown again.

Masks used to be frightening things.

The demon at the carnival.

The armed bank robber.

The Hallowe'en clown.

Now the virus is airborne—it's frightening because it is invisible.

Outside, masked people are now frightened of unmasked people.

Outside, unmasked people want to convince masked people to remove their masks.

It is safest not to reply, not to breathe, it is safest to walk away.

It is safest to now disregard all the social rules which have been so carefully learned.

It is safest to become reclusive and refuse to go outside at all.

I exhale in relief because for now it is perfectly acceptable to stop trying so hard to make friends.

Mask

When the ghost speaks there are gaps.

She censors her words using overlayers of gasps, as if other words are hidden in clumps of air:

I   a daughter.   to grow up.
                         Meet a boy   no   A girl
because I don't   at all.   secrets   with
no picnic   .   ever   complete   and don't
go   don't care   becauSe all I liKe   is
drawing   .   don't   .   want to play
five cats and one day a dog/wolf. And   who's kind   who's
kind?
            .   care it's   coMe Away   to eat
on the moor   and   . Seek   hiding   talK   .

The ghost's words disappear under false breath. Her past as well as mine has disappeared along with all the things I've done wrong and forgotten.

Mask

My final assessment appointment with Doctor X was three days ago, on Skype because of the lockdown. She's assessing me to find out if I'm autistic. The appointment happened in the front room of our home. Door closed. Headphones on. Focus.

I'll get her conclusion next week.

The ghost's shoulders stiffen. She hears my thoughts. Or feels them.

Perhaps she hid beside the closed door and saw me talking to Doctor X through a computer screen.

An odd conversation through glass with no reflections might be the kind of thing a ghost might watch.

Mask

—to reflect / seek similarities / mirror.

I wonder if my mum and any of my three brothers are autistic. I wonder if my dad was autistic. I wonder if Morgan is autistic.

I'll find out for certain if I am or not, next week. I've done diagnostic tests and ticked boxes. I've written pages about my childhood memories. I've completed questionnaires. My mum has answered questions and written a statement. Morgan has written a statement. I've filled out more questionnaires. Had conversations about childhood. Another test with scenarios and behaviours and opinions and layers of words and language designed to find gaps, lacks, empty spaces.

Tests to examine the things which don't fit quite the way they're expected to.

The wrong things.

I don't want to talk about the wrong things. I don't want to think about them.

Each morning, I forget them over and over again.

I'm trying to understand why no matter where I am or who I'm with, I'm lonely. I like being on my own, or being quiet and solitary, but loneliness is a painful emotion.

I wonder if Doctor X is autistic.

When I find out the answer about whether I am autistic or not, I don't want to speak about it because to hear a response could make me even lonelier.

I wonder if the ghost is autistic.

Mask

—to avoid seeing, or remove from sight.

The diagnostic tests for autism are based on data gathered from autistic boys. Girls have to present severe behavioural problems or intellectual disabilities to meet the criteria. Autistic girls and women are under-diagnosed. They have learned how to mask. How to appear. It takes a highly experienced specialist to be able to assess women who have spent a lifetime, masking.

—adapting, to adopt behaviours in order to fit in.

Women learn throughout their lifetime how to appear.
Have autistic women learned how to appear to appear?

Mask

—to redact / censor / hide the face.

The teenage ghost has been shouting, I think. She won't look at me because she doesn't want me to see the hurt under the anger under her hair-mask.

She doesn't want me to see her naked ghost-face.

Mask

Appearing   is   irrelevant   if no one
                sees   behind the   .

Mask

I've told very few people I'm having this assessment. Other people's voices, while well-intentioned, echo with unknowing which reverberates with my own doubts:

'But you're clever. Imaginative.'

'There's a highly sensitive personality type—you're more that, aren't you?'

'But you're such a good teacher, a brilliant writer, you've even got a PhD.'

'I think you're the opposite of autistic. Is that an empath?'

Recent studies suggest autistic people aren't lacking in empathy, but have too much empathy.

High sensitivity is also indicated.

Limited interests.

Sensory overwhelm.

Overload.

Difficulty with small talk.

Whether I'm autistic or not, I'm sensitive to people discussing whether I seem autistic or not.

I'm sensitive to the assumptions many people, including myself, make about autistic people.

I'm sensitive to all the things I do wrong.

I have listed all the reasons I might be autistic in my responses to the questionnaires and statements written during the assessment.

Pages of unrepeatable events and complicated relationships and misunderstandings and the wrong things I keep trying to forget.

I am relieved that after writing the wrong things down and discussing them with Doctor X I am still able to wake up and forget them.

All the same, this whole assessment might be an expensive mistake.

Mask

—a pointless investigation into overactive empathy and the permanence of loneliness.

Mask

The ghost measures language against its absence.

Miss	but			never	ask
hate	being	.	**A**		Secret

Keeper.

I close my eyes and examine the ghost's memories. She's been shouting at my dad because she is a teenager and he is her dad. Now she feels guilty about all the words she's shouted at him, because he is dead.

She was fourteen in 1986. She is still fourteen in 2021 and my dad has been suddenly dead for over six years.

She is stuck, aged fourteen. From the corner of the room she stares down at me through her tangled hair.

She's been shouting about all the wrong things she couldn't say.

Mask

I can see the ghost's blue eyes faintly through her hair and they are damp with tears.

<pre>
          I   MeAn   I hate it
   so   Scared   when I   rip   up
tug   tear   Keep   secrets.
</pre>

The ghost has wrapped her arms around herself.

She's so frightened of keeping secrets, she's trembling.

Mask

I wake, remembering my dad is dead.

I used to talk to him about the wrong things I couldn't usually talk about.

Remembering he's dead is like curled grey leaves, like the cruelty of ivory.

Mask

Before I open my eyes I wake in this double bed beside Morgan.

I roll over and put my arm around her waist.

Her murmur comes as a reply. A breath.

Silence.

Outside the window birds sing up the sun. A tūī with its double voicebox. Another tūī wakes, and another. They talk in overlayers of percussion. Click clack a ooo cluk.

We are lucky we don't have to go outside today and dawn is still the brightest thing.

These birds seem so much louder than ever before.

I touch Morgan's spine with my lips as I whisper 'love you, sweetheart.'

She murmurs, 'Mmm... love you too. Coffee...'

Smiling, I wake in a double bed with Morgan who loves me almost as much as she loves coffee.

What on earth would I do, without her.

I forget this wrong thought and hold her for a while longer, cradling warmth.

When I have forgotten everything I've done wrong, I try to forget how it feels to keep secrets.

As the birds sing louder the white walls become lighter.

The ghost grows paler as she disappears into daylight.

Mask

It's frightening to think I might have worn a mask my whole life.

It's frightening to think I might want to take it off. It's frightening to think there's no mask, that I just don't fit. That I have always been lonely for no reason other than I was born lonely.

I might take off my mask.

I might take off my mask and find my own naked face.

I might take off my naked face and find that behind it there is only a ghost.

Fourteen Words for Loneliness

Despane– The loneliness of feeling misunderstood, unloved or unheard by someone who used to understand, love or listen.

Starn– Craving something or someone to be there but knowing it's/they're not. Wanting to bite something.

Youache– Where a specific person is missed and only their physical presence will cure the ache of missing them.

Ignornly– The kind of loneliness that other people notice, but don't mention to the person they think is lonely. Their expression shows sympathy, but also a little wariness, as if loneliness could be contagious.

Solilone– A type of melancholia experienced while gazing at a wide-skied landscape. A longing for strangeness, for the unreal or the surreal to appear.

Idealone– A hankering for an imagined scenario—where it's the idea of the situation that causes the loneliness. For example, the 'ideal' of the perfect friend sitting opposite on the sofa, laughing over wine and confessions and saying all of the right things.

Achiposs– The ache of missing out on experiencing something beautiful, because it is impossible.

Disampty– Where the immediate environment is problematic – usually in practical ways. The rubbish split all over the floor, the smoke alarm is going off, work is waiting, the clock is ticking, the umbrella's broken, it's lashing with rain and there's no one else around.

Crowdsad– Felt while around many other people. Crying while walking along streets crammed with strangers, feeling unable to speak during a burbling conversation in which others are talking loudly and not leaving any gaps.

Feartrap– when alone, overactive fears producing images of other people becoming monstrous.

Priclash– Keeping emotions or secrets private while desperately wanting to let them out.

Xiley– The loneliness of ears: usually during unexpected silence. For example, when any music player suddenly ceases to work and refuses to be fixed.

Lonmyth– the belief that no one cares / is interested, without any effort to allow people to care or show that they're interested.

Uncharm– When you realise that no matter where you go, everywhere and everyone looks almost exactly the same.

Unstructured Collisions

Pretending everything is ordinary means everything ordinary can get done. I wake early and drink strong coffee before applying lipstick and attending a Zoom work meeting for three hours. Oblongs on screen. Watching multiple faces. Talking. Not-talking. Blank screen. Gone.

I wander outside for a walk. Moving away from pavements, seeking out parks and trees and grass. Climbing a hill beside a playing field until I'm breathless and high enough to inhale the wind.

The sea is a blue horizon above rows of urban buildings. All the windows of Wellington gleam under this winter sunlight.

I don't think about the diagnosis I was given yesterday.

There are so many other things to think about. Morgan. Lockdown. Inequalities. Laundry. The pandemic. Tidying my desk. The two growing kittens we've recently adopted. Upsetting global politics. The mental health of the students I teach. Online shopping. Our families in Scotland and Wales and England. Closed borders. So many Covid deaths. The women in Afghanistan. Where to buy milk. All the people hidden behind the walls, under the rooftops in this vast urban sprawl of houses and flats. The dark shadows of the trees on that other hill, over there. The tabby cat I passed on my way here. The birds in those trees. The eggs in nests. Are there nests, yet? Or is it still too cold? Imaginary chicks growing inside imaginary eggs. The chicks' brains filled with imaginary nightmares about hatching. The crack in an imaginary eggshell.

Cracks in walls, in roads, in windowpanes. The sharpness of all broken edges.

Thinking about other things that aren't this diagnosis is not as easy as inhaling and exhaling the wind. But it is nearly as easy as imagining the nightmares of unhatched chicks.

I return home to make notes on student stories and run a two hour Zoom class. Student faces in oblongs. I make sure everyone is kind to each other, that everyone hears useful ideas about how to develop their characters, how to build a fictional world and inhabit it. I talk about narrative modes and recite the most brilliant quotes from each of their stories—showing them if they give their writing drafts energy and thought and time, they could become strong.

Their smiles are genuine but their eyes seem so tired.

Once everyone has gone blank on the screen, I close my laptop to end the working day.

And now I can let myself think about yesterday's diagnosis. In this same room. This desk. The same window showing the roses and trees behind my computer screen.

Only I can't think properly, because my thoughts are too fast.

Doctor X's unfrowning-unsmiling face on the screen. Reading glasses. Her soft-textured cardigan. Voice calm, focussed on giving information. Frank and direct. 'I'll give you a brief verbal confirmation today. The report will follow.'

Memories flash flash flash like bright noise. Flash Christmas lights. Red-green smell. Smells of pepper, lavender, baked potatoes, porridge.

Her voice, 'You've been diagnosed with giftedness and ASD.'

I'm autistic.

Memory-smells. Flash school uniform. Flute sound.

I remember my autistic cousin as a beautiful toddler running around a large empty room, chasing sound.

She said, 'Some people find it more helpful to think of it as autism spectrum difference, rather than autism spectrum disorder.' She explained that Asperger's wasn't used as a diagnostic term any more, but that's what my diagnosis would have once been called. She kept talking. I kept silent. I nodded a lot. At the end she said, 'Do you have questions?'

'Not right now.' I replied. 'I'll do some reading.'

'I'll send you a reading list,' she said. 'There's a very small support group too, but that's difficult as you don't drive. We won't meet till we're at Covid level one, probably. And who knows when that will be.'

I thanked her for her time, made arrangements for payment, and the screen turned blank.

Flash of red and purple fuchsia flowers.

Nettles. Thistles. Thorns.

On my phone I attempt to read academic papers about autism and the words blur. I try to find out about giftedness and can't find anything useful. Do these two things run in parallel or crash into each other like wonky steam trains? As I can't focus on finding the right questions to seek answers to, I worry about talking. I worry about the assumptions and confusion and opinions of other people if I decide to mention this diagnosis. Misconception—autism equals Rain Man. Misconception—autism equals no empathy. I know all the misconceptions. But I don't know how to explain them to other people, because I don't know how to explain myself to other people.

From the sofa, Morgan is watching TED talks. I'm sitting by the back door listening to the night birds calling each other. I half-hear the sound of a passionate academic's voice. 'Some studies show not a lack of empathy, but a difference in how empathy is experienced.' I half-hear the voice saying. 'We might, more simply, use the word 'neurodiverse'.' And yet another: 'If you have only met one autistic person, you have only met one autistic person. With neurodiversity, no two minds are the same.'

There aren't any words in my mouth.

Morgan's getting a glass of water. She's wearing her blue t-shirt which says 'You Wouldn't Understand: It's a Morgan Thing'. Standing behind her at the sink, I untangle the back of her long hair, teasing out the strands with my thumbs.

I say, 'I'm scared you'll stop loving me because of this diagnosis.'

She replies, 'Don't be silly. Thanks for sorting my bedhead.'

'But what if how you think of me changes? What if you begin to see me in a different way?' I smooth her hair with my palm.

She turns around and her eyes soften as she looks at me, 'But I already know exactly who you are. I've always known.'

I smile.

'Haven't I?' she says, wrapping her arms around me.

I lean my forehead against hers.

Even though no two minds are the same, we two are extremely similar.

I think she's very likely to be autistic too. We've discussed it many times.

We sleep in a bedful of crowded and unremembered dreams.

I wake feeling small, wanting to be picked up and carried by a giant eagle.

Needing to walk away from this feeling, I go outside. Wearing a mask I walk along pavements. Strangers wearing masks are tall shadows. The inside of my head is full of bright noise; I miss all the eagles I've known. I miss my eagle dad. I miss my eagle mum and three eagle brothers. I miss my eagle friend Tim who I've known since 1989. I made friends with Tim by following him around till he liked me. I miss eagle Jay who wore feathers and bones in his hair. I miss Eagle Paul who I've known since 2000. I worked with Paul for twelve years. He must have learned to like me slowly, and so did eagle Edd, who was my counsellor and then after a break, became my friend. I miss eagle Sophie and eagle Andy who I've known since around 1995. They were my neighbours in Brighton—a five-storey Regency house with two tiny flats on each floor. No lift. We lived on the top floors, hanging out of the windows and watching miniature people in the streets below. We stalked in and out of each other's rooms, discussing relationship breakups, lost drugs, problems with mail theft. We celebrated birthdays, studied courses, started jobs.

But even when I lived among eagles, I felt lonely. Though I've felt lonely my whole life, it's been getting worse as I get older. I've been trying to tell myself it's all right. That all kinds of people feel permanently lonely. The difference is I'll *say* I'm lonely, knowing there are consequences. Knowing one of these consequences is that most people avoid lonely people.

Via email, I receive a resource list including recommended books and academic papers about autism. Each bold title is a dark rock on the page. How do I get hold of books while we're in lockdown? Library. No. Post. Are books classified as essential items? Which website? I try two bookshops online, but they haven't got these titles. Another library is recommended by google. Are borders closed to books, as well as people? I can't tell which country it's in.

One paper I can't even open mentions something about unstructured thoughts in its Abstract. Is that where my mind goes when facing too many things all at once? Into an abstract place; the internet as a vast network of unstructured collisions. The whole world is a vast network of unstructured collisions. Collusions? Feeling too small today; I draw tiny birds on huge sheets of black paper. In the sky there are no other humans.

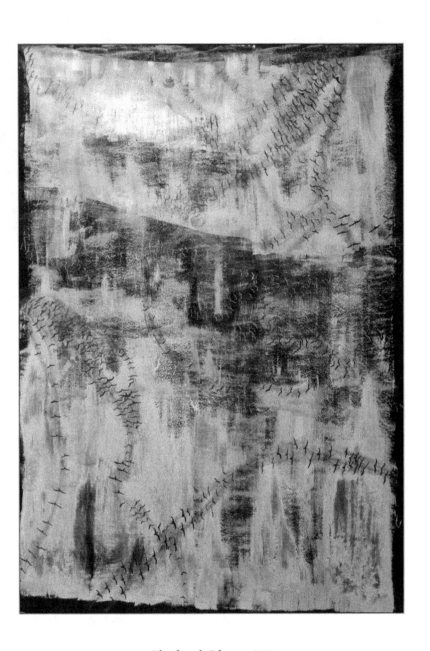

Flock of Ghosts VII

I wake full of bright noise. I wake remembering misunderstandings. Remembering trying and failing to ever be able to do maths. Remembering how to walk away. Remembering unkindnesses, remembering how not to care. Remembering that even some of the eagles I miss were mean at times. Does missing them make them seem kinder than they were? Memory is a filter. A camera lens. In the past there were also eagles who were cruel. I don't want to have ever been ripped at or clawed. If I don't remember it, it didn't happen. Did anyone who was mean or cruel to me ever say sorry? I don't remember which ones said sorry. I'll adjust the lens and apply a sorry-filter so I can remember their apologies. I can imagine just about anything. If I imagine it often enough and vividly enough, it'll get transferred from short term to long term memory.

Apologetic eagles are bedraggled creatures.

Putting on a mask, I wander outside and walk and walk and walk. It's hard to know what other people are thinking when there's only their eyes. Everyone's too unpredictable. What filter do they have over their eyes when they look at each other? Today I've got a frightened-filter. Some of them do too.

I'm not sure I know instinctively who to trust. I'm not sure I trust myself to recognise unkindness before it intensifies to become cruelty. In the past, I stayed in a damaging relationship for far too long. In the even more distant past I got into a violent situation because I thought I could trust a stranger.

The strangers in masks are too close, too unpredictable, too lurching. My thoughts are mirroring them and becoming too unpredictable, too lurching.

I rush back home to Morgan who I completely trust.

She's sitting by the fire typing an email to her sister. She's got classical music playing, to keep her calm while she waits and hopes for immunity, two weeks after having both Covid jabs. 'Hey sweetheart, good walk?'

'It was all right. Not as good as I thought it would be.' I grin at her, as this is a joke we often share when describing our new stripy kittens and their various disappointments. 'How are you?'

'Mm. Yup... fine.' Her eyes flicker towards her screen. She's still half in her email. I make us a coffee, go into the other room and open my work laptop.

I try to do some marking but can't concentrate yet because my thoughts are too fast. So I make us beans on toast instead and feel grateful for lockdown throwing all routines out of whack apart from simple and practical things. I'm feeling a bit numb so I get a scourer out of the cupboard and run the hot tap. I scrub the metal kitchen sink as if it were possible to make it shine like a mirror. The water isn't hot enough for my hands to feel it yet so I turn it up until the sink is steaming and my hands become pink. Real things will save me from disintegrating. The sink still isn't shining, but I scrub the counter beside it, then the cooker. I can't feel my arms, so I wipe down the cupboards with cleaning spray which smells of oranges until they feel real again. I prep for the next evening class and email some handouts out. To feel my legs I go down the steps to the tiny room under the house and do the laundry. I stay up late, making my shoulders hurt till they feel solid and real, hunched over my laptop marking student stories and poems.

Some of the stories are instinctive. Others are odd and fearful. No two are the same.

It's strange to examine stories and poems through the filter of a grade.

To give words a number.

At night-time I stand in the garden with a freezing southerly gale blowing all around me.

I'm trying to feel the ground as a solid thing.

Thoughts blow through my hair as it tangles around my head, blindfolds my eyes, covers my face.

I'm trying to force my bright-noise thoughts to slow down so I can see them and make them stop.

Colours: orange pink neon blue sunsets spreading across the Irish sea. Scents of clover and pine. Sitting on the pavement opposite my empty ex-home in Brighton, hiding my tears with a scarf. Walking in Scotland with my dad as he stopped me by gripping my arm and pointing at an adder snake curled on the path. Being in Queenstown with Morgan looking at a view of perfect silver water and perfect purple mountains and a perfect pale blue sky. Making watercolour paintings of geranium plants at secondary school. My dad was oddly hypersensitive to the smell of geraniums but he praised my paintings.

Stockpiling antidepressants and taping them and a razor blade to the back of a dresser drawer in Brighton. The underside of the brick archways of Victorian viaducts. Sharing chips with Morgan and the gulls on the beach at Island Bay. My mum teaching me to knit by showing my hands what to do. Earthquake-prone stickers on locked Newtown doors. Dark cliffs and my three brothers climbing jagged rocks. Kissing Morgan for the first time in a hotel room in York. Slate roof tiles crashing down in winter storms. Archaeological digs with skeletons in rows, jaws open. The heady flavour of Manuka honey, tasted for the very first time. The grey-green ocean flecked with waves, kelpies, the manes of white horses. Walking along Lyall Bay with Morgan dragging the trolley she'd wheeled to the airport to meet me and my broken blue suitcase when I first landed in New Zealand.

Standing here in our garden now, trying to feel the ground. I hunch my shoulders like a giant bird. My hair is full of memories, blown all around my face. My hair becomes dark feathers, tangled by this icy wind that's travelled all the way from Antarctica.

Our firewood delivery arrives as a heap on the pavement. Morgan and I shift it to the side of our narrow house and stack it along the fence. We work well together, me lifting, wheeling and dropping, her dividing and stacking. Once it's all done, my back twists, threatening to spasm.

It is best not to panic, or the spasm gets worse and fast. Forced to lie flat, my head fills with fast-thoughts about being unable to move, so I try to think of other things. I lie on our bed watching memory pictures flash flash flash across the white ceiling. Ivy leaves. School desks with lids on hinges. A butterfly sticker over a coat hook with my name on it. Moss. Sea thrift. Forget-me-nots. Daisies, petals pinched off, 'Love me or love me not.' I try not to remember the other times my back's gone out. Other times when my body has had enough of my fast head and made me stop whatever I'm doing too much of and forced me to be still. A fifth floor flat in Brighton, lying on the floor crying about the doctor telling me I had to take at least seven days off work and knowing I wouldn't get paid sick leave. Love me or love me not how will I pay our council tax bill? Nine years later, lying on the floor in a ground floor flat in Brighton believing I couldn't take seven days off work because I wouldn't get paid sick leave and no one else knew how to do my job. Love me or love me not how will I cover our electricity and gas bills and how will the students get the right exam papers at the right time? I remember and forget and remember.

I stare at the white paper lampshade on the bedroom ceiling and try to think of soft things. Rose petals. Haiku poems. Thistledown. Marshmallow sweets. Bubble wrap. The tiny chunks of fake snow in snow globes. Bath foam. My eyes fill with tears as I lie here remembering all the cats I've ever loved. Cyrus. Pussy. Toby. Biba. Muffin. Wicca. Zoe. Meg. Pudding. Minky. Mottle. The two Furies. Kitty. Puck. Madam Sin. Charlie. Kenny. Morgan's girl Gwennie, an elderly ginger beauty who lived with us when I first arrived in New Zealand. And the cats we have now. Boy, a part time stray who's still visiting us for a couple of hours of food and love each night. The stripy kittens: Danu. Toto. Born on the last day of 2020. I lie here remembering all the human friends I never fell out with, but don't hear from any more.

I miss all the cats so much.

There were bullies in my first job in the produce department at the local supermarket. The manager was the worst but she also enlisted help from two other staff, closer to my age. One of them was recently bereaved and trying to impress the other, older one. I've never thought of them as bullies, till now. But you don't lock a sixteen-year-old in a walk-in fruit and vegetable fridge and leave her there if you're not mean.

At nine thirty, one of them said a box of tomatoes needed to go on the trolley to be taken up to the shop floor. I went into the walk-in fridge to get them. The door was slammed shut behind me. I was between the tall metal rows of shelves, tomatoes on one side of my head, grapes on the other. Through the frosted window in the fridge door, a blurry face looked in, eyes gleaming. The lock clicked and the face disappeared. I approached the door, knowing it wouldn't open but checking it just in case, with a slight shove.

I looked out of the fridge window at the vague shape of the empty ramps and storage area. The lift door was shut. They would have gone back up to the shop floor with the trolley. The shop uniform was scratchy nylon, a green pinny over an orange overall. My leather shoes were thick soled, but I was wearing thin tights. The air was icy but I didn't believe they were murderers.

After some time had passed, a blurred face looked in the window with a lopsided grin. I pushed at the door, but it was still locked. The grin laughed and disappeared again. I was cold, but how quickly would I get *too* cold? My watch told me I'd just missed my ten-minute tea break.

I didn't want to speak or shout.

Deciding that I wouldn't speak meant I was able to remain completely calm.

While I waited for them to let me out again, I ate a punnet of cherries. If I got caught eating by one of the managers, I'd get sacked for thieving. So I stood with my back to the fridge door, swallowed the cherry stones and hid the empty punnet beneath a full one.

My lips still tasted of cherries when they finally returned and opened the door.

One of them said, 'The manager's been asking where you were.'

The other jumped in. 'You're in trouble. You're to get upstairs, right now. You should have been on the shop floor all morning.'

My watch said it was mid-day, so my shift was over. I went down the ramp past the lifts and along the corridor to the locker room. I got changed into my jeans and sweatshirt and returned to the ramp. I walked along the side corridor and let myself out of the trade door.

I went down to the shore and kicked at stones. I didn't talk for the rest of the day. Not till I had to. As soon as I spoke, I felt upset.

For weeks afterwards I thought I still had cherry stones in my guts and a blossoming cherry tree would grow inside me.

I remember the wind, last night in the garden, blowing my memories through my hair. Changing direction.

Kindness.

In Brighton my eagle friend Jac gave me an enamel butterfly brooch for my birthday one year. I have it with me here in New Zealand, in a small white cardboard box. It's a tiny red thing, the colour of my wedding dress. My eagle friend Ros sent me a pirate hot water bottle in the post. I'd recently left Brighton and was freezing through the winter looking after empty holiday cottages at Kintyre. My eagle tutor

Catherine quoted from my first published short story in a book she was writing a chapter for. She said she wanted to be the first person to ever write about me. My eagle friend Cliff let me attend his poetry classes and also made time to read my draft poems. I met these kind people because I'd gone to creative writing night classes after work. If I hadn't written stories, I'd never have met them.

To me, writing is speaking. An attempt to be heard. To be more open.

But right now I can't remember how to make friends.

Doctor X said something about that when she diagnosed me.

What was it she said?

Everyone in New Zealand is friendly, but I don't seem to be able to get past the surface.

I can't remember how friendships start and keep going.

What I did or what they did, to make it work.

How long it takes.

I talk to my family on Skype and don't tell them about the autism diagnosis because I don't have the right words in my mouth. I haven't seen them in person for more than three years. My mum's tabby, Fliss, is on the table beside her in her oblong on the screen as a swirl of black and grey stripes. My three brothers look back at me from their oblongs while I ask about their lives, their jobs, families, and what's going on with Covid in Scotland.

In my middle brother's oblong, his cat Fudge meows and climbs up his chest.

'Everything's quiet here,' I say, 'You know what lockdown's like— you were in it far longer. Well, quiet apart from the kittens. They're vandals.'

Stroking Fudge, he laughs and says, 'Kittens are for life, not just for lockdown.'

'They've started going outside and exploring.'

My youngest brother's daughter comes into his oblong and we all fill our oblongs with love heart emojis to make her sweet face laugh. While everyone talks about my oldest brother's new rescue dog, Duncan, their oblongs are full of the pale daylight of the Northern Hemisphere. It's night-time here and my oblong looks like a black and white Victorian photograph. I re-angle the desk lamp and cast too much light. Bleach out my skin, shadow my eyes. The only thing missing is some ectoplasm made of net. I move the lamp back again.

Our kittens are in the other room with Morgan, asleep by the fire. While my brothers are talking I'm thinking of their pets and wishing I could sit quietly stroking them. I'm thinking of our kittens and the cars in our street. I'm thinking of the grey whippet next door. I'm thinking of all the things the kittens should be more scared of. I'm wondering how long it takes cats to learn fear. I'm wishing they didn't have to.

My middle brother's laughing at our niece and sending her a monkey emoji.

She sends him a balloon and a cupcake and a violin.

I love seeing them all laugh. When did my family stop being afraid of Covid? They've all been vaccinated for a while now.

My oldest brother sends our niece an acrobat.

I send a vampire.

She sends a circus tent and a hot dog and rain.

I remember my own fear for them, more than their fear for themselves. Perhaps I don't listen well enough. It's hard to listen and look at them in their oblongs, simultaneously.

My mum says, 'I'm meeting a friend down at Soleburn soon. What are you doing today, all of you? Jess, you'll be off to bed.'

I nod and send a crescent moon emoji.

My middle brother says, 'We'll probably go to the farm shop for cake and coffee.'

My youngest brother says, 'I'm going for a run and then dropping my daughter off at her friend's house.'

My eldest brother says, 'I'm heading north for a dive.'

It's like watching people I love on television but not acting—being themselves. I wish I knew when, even roughly, I'll be able to see them outside of these oblongs. Next year? The year after? Five years? Ten?

My eldest brother takes a sip of pixelated coffee while my middle brother asks, 'Are you and Morgan doing OK, Jess?'

I say, 'We're scared the kittens will run away.'

My mum shakes her head and blurs orange and green through her oblong.

'They won't,' she says. 'They'll come back to you.'

Fifteen Words for Loneliness

Despane– The loneliness of feeling misunderstood, unloved or unheard by someone who used to understand, love or listen.

Starn– Craving something or someone to be there but knowing it's/they're not. Wanting to bite something.

Youache– Where a specific person is missed and only their physical presence will cure the ache of missing them.

Ignornly– The kind of loneliness that other people notice, but don't mention to the person they think is lonely. Their expression shows sympathy, but also a little wariness, as if loneliness could be contagious.

Solilone– A type of melancholia experienced while gazing at a wide-skied landscape. A longing for strangeness, for the unreal or the surreal to appear.

Idealone– A hankering for an imagined scenario—where it's the idea of the situation that causes the loneliness. For example, the 'ideal' of the perfect friend sitting opposite on the sofa, laughing over wine and confessions and saying all of the right things.

Achiposs– The ache of missing out on experiencing something beautiful, because it is impossible.

Disampty– Where the immediate environment is problematic – usually in practical ways. The rubbish split all over the floor, the smoke alarm is going off, work is waiting, the clock is ticking, the umbrella's broken, it's lashing with rain and there's no one else around.

Crowdsad– Felt while around many other people. Crying while walking along streets crammed with strangers, feeling unable to speak during a burbling conversation in which others are talking loudly and not leaving any gaps.

Feartrap– when alone, overactive fears producing images of other people becoming monstrous.

Priclash– Keeping emotions or secrets private while desperately wanting to let them out.

Xiley– The loneliness of ears: usually during unexpected silence. For example, when any music player suddenly ceases to work and refuses to be fixed.

Lonmyth– the belief that no one cares / is interested, without any effort to allow people to care or show that they're interested.

Uncharm– When you realise that no matter where you go, everywhere and everyone looks almost exactly the same.

Upwrench– The rational side – loneliness needs to be felt and solitude is needed even if it's not always comfortable. Letting loneliness come, but giving it a time limit: not wallowing.

Noise and Quiet

The pandemic is a loud thing. It sends people home and makes us all fearful. It fills the home with screens full of work and frequent television announcements. It fills the eyes with news apps to scroll through, it fills the brain with information to fret over.

The pandemic is a loud thing. As soon as this lockdown ends, social media will again flood with loud photos of reunited parents and children, grandparents and babies, reunited siblings, nieces and nephews.

The pandemic is a loud thing. The reunited-close-friends photographs will then start appearing to be scrolled through. Online bullying will become even more brutal, more obvious. Anger has got to come out somewhere, and screens act as shields. Death-threats express unpunctuated violence within 280 characters. Apparitions of cruelty, repeated as language on a loop. Online conversations fuelled by fear transform too easily into violence.

There will be no photos of people making new friends. During a pandemic, people want to reunite with the people they already know, already love, already trust.

The pandemic is a loud thing that also brings quietness. It's impossible to think about the future, to make promises, to plan ahead. For a long time, my loud thoughts have involved telling myself I'm not trying hard enough, or am not good enough, or have done something wrong, or that I'm thinking or speaking in all the wrong ways.

The pandemic brings quietness. During the first lockdown it was such a relief, to have a break from trying so hard to connect with other people, and failing. It made me think a lot, about how much brighter the world might seem if I could just allow myself to stop trying.

The pandemic brings quietness. Without having to try and fail at small talk, without meeting people in confusing groups in loud gasping places, without going to bright work parties and leaving again because I don't know how to join in conversations, without meeting someone one-to-one and enjoying the conversation but not knowing what to do next so doing nothing, without giving up doing nothing and convincing myself to try and fail all over again, I can finally exhale. I can look at social media without making a sound and be no more than a witness to other conversations. I can switch off and go blank.

Blank as a ghost.

The pandemic brings quietness. Quietness allows thoughts to slow down enough to see them. The slow thoughts about loneliness I had during the first lockdown prompted me to get the autism assessment done. I'd always wondered, but the relief of not having to communicate with others gave me time to think and read more about autism. But is everything now too quiet? Sometimes. I feel haunted when the things I can't say get stuck in my body. My own ghost enters the room, telling me not to keep secrets.

The pandemic has made the days and nights more silent. Silence is a relief. A reason to finally breathe. Leaving Brighton and being transient, then falling in love and my dad's death and flying away, migrating—these are all loud things. But landing? Landing is a quiet thing when there's no requirement to go outside. It is safest to stay at home. Just safe Morgan and me and our safe hands. A safe garden. A safe home. Our safe hearts and a safe sleep and safe waking. It's safely silent, after all the noise which has gone before.

And now I've made some noise. I've been diagnosed with autism. Love me. Don't love me not. Please keep loving me.

Of course she will. We are the same.

But what if we're not?

Morgan's decided to get assessed as well.

'But what if I'm not autistic too,' she says. 'Will you still love me?'

I laugh. 'Whatever someone else says you are or aren't, you're my best one. I've always wanted a Morgan of my own. Nothing changes.'

I understand why she'd worry; we've always valued our similarities. Many of the first conversations we had were all about experiences we'd had which were similar. How annoyed some of our ex-partners had been because we were too silent or self-sufficient. What we see when we retreat into our own minds. What kinds of poetry and literature, songs and paintings, colours or sounds or images we like best. When we first started talking via email, we'd send each other imaginary gifts.

'For you—three eyelashes from a spider who's just discovered crimson mascara.'

'For you—the sound of an eggshell shattering and the first chirp of a flamingo chick.'

Now we've been together for several years, we often say exactly the same thing at exactly the same time and have no idea what prompted the thought in the first place.

I wake and lie in bed for a while with my eyes shut, letting my thoughts slow. I'm trying to see what my brain is trying to do with all this fast thinking. I'm remembering my life all over again—in fragments, out of linear order. My brain is trying to refocus each memory with a lens twist, showing images with a slightly different filter. The lens reshuffles my life through the filter of being autistic. This is solitary, because it has to be. Other people might just about understand the word 'Asperger's' even though this word isn't used in diagnostic assessments any more. 'High functioning' and 'low functioning' are also now considered judgemental terms. But they were once, at least, familiar. Now I have no language to explain myself with. Maybe I can get away without talking about autism or ASD or Asperger's at all, even though I hate keeping secrets. No one knows about giftedness so it's probably best to never even mention it. I'm not sure what I'm gifted at anyway because I'm only good at two things: writing and drawing. I'm either terrible at, or not interested in, everything else.

She said something about friendships that I've been trying to remember. I remember it now—she said that friendships between autistic people can look quite different to neurotypical friendships. That autistic friends might only see each other once a year, or less, and that's often enough.

I wonder about all the people I used to call friends. People like talking about themselves and I prefer listening to speaking. Perhaps they were beside me because I was easy to talk to. The curve of my ear, an echoing seashell. Do they remember me and know I still think about them?

I don't hear from them anymore. And I don't automatically think to reach out or make contact. Do we all only see whatever's directly in front of our eyes?

At night time I go for a walk and there are no other humans.

I look for stars but they're hidden by clouds. In the sky there are no other humans. I keep looking upwards.

Walking along damp pavements I reach to touch each tree's leaves with my fingertips.

There's a cracking sound beneath my boot.

Tiny snails slowly cross the pavements.

I pick each one up and move it onto the grass verge.

There are so many snails. It takes me a long time to get home.

Can't wake up properly. My brain is too busy sorting my memories out with their new filters and I can't even connect the images because they're in the illogical order of a half-dream. I keep remembering people being mean to me. I used to ignore mean things people did but they're suddenly painful to think about, with this new autistic filter. There are a lot of mean memories for my brain to work through. I wish it would give me some kind of control, or even the illusion of control. But there isn't any. My brain is starting to slow down. I look at photographs on Facebook of people I used to call friends. All of these photographs are of other places, other times. Were they just nearby people, who talked back to me when I was beside them and forgot me when I was away from their eyes?

People I went to school with have posted photo collages of our teenage parties. I recognise the locations; some are even at my mum's house. I'm not in any of them. This is a relief in some ways, as I would have been drunk and I don't really want to see evidence of this. But my absence also makes me question if I was really there, talking, dancing, laughing with them.

Or if I appeared and disappeared to them, as an apparition.

I don't have my own photographs any more, because of forgetting to take that precious box of photographs from Brighton. I can't remember all the memories that have been lost.

Have I ever really known anyone? Has anyone ever really known me?

I feel like I've been a ghost all my life and not realised it till now.

Can't talk or I'll cry. Half-want to talk. Half-don't. Can't find words.

I'm not fully awake yet. I keep thinking about how much easier it would be to stop talking altogether and remain blissfully silent.

I wrote fifteen new words / definitions of different kinds of loneliness about nine years ago and gave them to an anchoress character in my third novel. I can add more definitions and types of loneliness to that list now. Perhaps this diagnosis will help me to simply accept that my loneliness is permanent.

Maybe one day I'll stop talking. I did this years ago for several days and nights, while I was at art college and had to force myself to start speaking again. While I was silent I was content. Happy. Confident. I occupied a parallel world where I could see everything going on around me, I felt untouchable and completely safe. But humans want other humans to speak. It seems impossible to be silent out of choice.

Loneliness is very different to being silent, or being alone, or solitary.

Here in New Zealand I talk to Morgan and we are also often silent together for long periods of time. I occasionally see her friends with her too; a long-term friend who lives down the road, her ex-PhD candidate and his equally clever partner, and a lovely young couple we talk to on Zoom if we can't see them in person. But I'm now realising that in general I talk to birds and animals and insects far more than I talk to other humans.

Especially cats. Always the cats. There's a white one down the road from here who I always whisper to, while I pass her. She blinks at me.

Cats like being talked to by humans as long as the voice is gentle.

If my friends are the cats, birds, the ocean, if my friends are stars, the sky, ferns, mountains, then I don't feel so lonely.

They listen and don't listen in ways I can understand.

I walk through Newtown and don't look at the masked human shadows who pass me.

When I don't speak, everything is alive and everything is more colourful.

The pigeons are my friends. The clouds are my friends. The wind is my friend.

I've never understood what people have meant in the past when they've said, 'You should show yourself the same compassion you show others.'

For the first time, I can see my own hurt. I can see the places hurt occurred. Primary school corridors. Secondary school classrooms, work staff rooms. In pubs and clubs and dark alleyways. In the rooms of all the homes I've ever had. I've always thought any pain I felt was my own fault for being too sensitive or not sensitive enough—for not recognising the warning signs or following my instincts until it was too late. I thought that hiding pain was the only thing to be done with it. Pretend hurt never happened at all, reach out to help others who clearly need it, and keep moving.

I gave all my compassion away to others, not realising it could flow inwards as well as outwards. But I'm beginning to feel compassionate towards myself for the first time.

When it can't be spoken, the language of hurt becomes the languages of the body. It is the language of throbs and scratches, aches and pulses. It is the languages of deep cracks and slipped discs, of knotted muscles, half-healed scars and undiagnosed breaks.

There is hurt everywhere. Individual pain is small in comparison. Here in Aotearoa New Zealand it's impossible not to be aware of deep collective pain. Here, as in many other colonised countries, indigenous languages were beaten out of children by English-speaking teachers. Language is lost, people are weakened and voices are silenced. This also happened in Wales, where I was born. And here, te reo Māori was stolen. Te reo is returning to this bicultural country, but painfully and slowly. Removing language is a violent and devastating way for one group of people to destroy another group of people.

Going outside, I wander down Adelaide Road. I walk around the curve of Island Bay. There are no other people on the pavements today. No human languages. The gulls are my friends. The heavy rain is my friend. The ocean is my friend. The gusting wind is my friend.

I wish I could have talked to my dad about autism, about him, about my mum, about me, my brothers, grandparents, the extended family.

We did talk. We talked about everything. We just didn't use labels.

Labels can be useful when they help to explain how something works.

I wish I could talk to him, now.

Silence is a protective scab.

I wander towards the centre of Wellington and don't look at the masked people who pass me.

The tūī and the blackbirds are my friends. The plants growing between paving stones are my friends. The breeze is my friend. The flax leaves are my friends.

When talking my mum on Skype, my laptop camera isn't working. She can't see my face, but I can see hers. Her flame red hair. Behind glasses, her bright blue eyes. Through the window, daylight. On the windowpanes, stickers of bird silhouettes.

She knew I was having the autism assessment because she needed to answer a lot of detailed questions about my childhood. I wanted her to be able to see me when I told her. But I don't want to wait till next time we talk.

I say, 'Because of lockdown, I had some Skype appointments. Children all need to be face-to-face. I've been diagnosed with two things—giftedness and autism.'

Though she can't see me, she looks directly into the camera and I hold her gaze with my unblinking eyes. My heart thuds, from speaking.

'It's probably not the cleverest thing I've done, being assessed for autism during a pandemic, while trapped on the other side of the world from my family. Morgan's being lovely, as always.'

My mum nods as if she can see me. But she can't. Her eyes look right into me. Or into an idea of me.

I say, 'I'm not sure what I'm gifted at. Maybe it's writing or my PhD. She had a look at some of my writing and art. So, let's talk about autism.'

We talk about it as if it is ordinary. We talk about other people in the family who probably are or were autistic. Mostly undiagnosed, apart from my cousin. Including her. Including my dad. Including my grandpa, who worried about my oversensitivity as a child. About how I'd cope with the world as an adult. We talk about misunderstandings, about small talk and uncomfortable social situations, about oddness and special interests. We talk about hyperactive empathy or the lack of empathy and we talk about the texture of people and their blurring shifting soft or jagged edges.

She tells me 'I've been burning the letters me and your father wrote to each other when we were teenagers. So soppy. I'm keeping one or two. I want them buried with me, unread. Have you got that?'

My heart aches for myself in the future, but I reply, 'Of course. I'll do whatever you want with them, as long as you tell me what that is.'

She nods, knowing I mean it.

I can't bear to think about her dying. I watch her face move in smudges and swirls of orange and pink pixels as she tells me about her GP appointment and about the man who came to fix her boiler. She tells me about going to the village to get eggs. How extraordinary all of these ordinary things seem to her now, after months of self-isolating and lockdowns.

'One day,' she says. 'One day you'll be here again. But when?'

'I still don't know.'

She returns to her day and I to the night as we close our screens.

After this conversation I wrap my arms around myself and think of the word 'familiarity'. It's the kind of word which hums, vibrates and echoes. It has the sound of guitar strings. I wonder if she's kept my dad's guitar. I think she has. Even across this distance of 11,489 miles and over three years of unanticipated separation there's a feeling of deep knowing. Of being deeply known.

I walk along pavements and don't look at the street names or the masked people who pass me. The tauhou and pigeons are my friends. The starlings are my cousins and the seagulls are my aunties and uncles. The piles of white-grey clouds are my brothers. The swerving wind is my mum.

I wake up crying, into a memory of being suicidal. I wake not knowing if I'm alive or dead.

258

Morgan rolls over and says, 'Come here, sweetheart. It's only a dream.' She wraps her arms around me and holds me close.

Am I only half-living, half-ghosting through borrowed time?

Am I only still alive because I love Morgan and because she loves me so much?

Am I more ghost than human?

The dawn birds are waking, calling in all of their languages.

I can feel scratches on my wrists but there's nothing there. I'm suddenly so cold.

Half-asleep, Morgan murmurs, 'Love you, baby. I've got you.'

There are songs stuck in my throat.

Am I more bird than ghost?

I stop crying because in this small white bedroom Morgan's wrapped all around me. She's warming me through with her strength.

Her arms are wings.

In YouTube videos there's a lot of talk about autistic people masking in order to appear the same as everyone else. This idea of 'masking' seems like acting or lying. A pretence. But this assumption doesn't seem fair—as everyone, autistic or not, adapts, acts, changes to fit different roles, different situations. Many people mask, en masse—but this isn't seen as being dishonest. Heterosexual mating rituals are a prime example of this. Hens and stags. Engagement parties, wedding lists, baby showers. Even vow renewals and divorce parties. They're practically scripted. Everyone has a part to play. Everyone is masking en masse, as a great big group.

But now everyone is individually masked because of the pandemic and we can only see each other's eyes. Until...

until one person in any group takes their mask off and glances around. This often happens in the evening classes I teach or attend. Once one person has unmasked and made eye contact, one after the other, everyone else in the group removes their masks. It's as if a conversation has been had and a group decision has been made.

In every situation where this happens, I think of Morgan. How afraid she is, of catching Covid. I care more about her fear, about her health, about her, than about group decisions. I'm often the only one in the room wearing a mask.

There's a psychological test that involves looking at black and white photographs of white people's eyes. There are four words for different emotions at each corner of the photograph. Pick only one. In the photographs the people look like they are masking their true feelings. The women wear thick eye makeup from the 1980s. The people in the photographs are actors.

They're acting the genuine emotion which people who are being tested are meant to find in their eyes.

Even psychological tests aren't trustworthy.

I read some more academic papers and this time, I focus. People who are neurodiverse can communicate fine with other people who are neurodiverse. People who are neurotypical can communicate fine with other people who are neurotypical. The problems must therefore come from miscommunication between neurodiverse and neurotypical brains.

Could it be a misunderstanding? Do humans look like one species, but are really two?

Morgan and I curl up together on the sofa and watch a nature documentary that demonstrates differences in the social behaviour of bonobo apes and chimps.

Morgan says, 'See—they look like chimps, but they're not.'

I nod. 'They seem cleverer and much less aggressive.'

On the screen, one climbs on top of another.

Morgan says, 'And they're really into sex.'

I wonder if roses speak the same language as flax flowers.

If leaves speak the same language as roots.

We blink at the kittens and the kittens blink back.

I love the lightness of their silence.

Do birds speak the same language as ghosts and do ghosts speak the same language as birds?

The people who've hurt me over the years were all masked in some way, until they showed me who they really were. I couldn't recognise their masks. To them it must have seemed easy, or right, to pretend to be kind, then suddenly change. Bullies also mask. They pretend to laugh and be friendly before trapping their prey. As hunters, birds are far more straightforward—they hover and swoop. Employees pretend to their managers they are capable and fair while bullying the employee below them. All politicians lie, or mask the truth. Most people don't know who anyone really is unless they've lived with them.

I don't know how to pretend. How to lie. I might have known, once. Not any more.

Maybe I'm not able to mask. Maybe I've never been able to.

I watch a documentary about dishonesty. A group of people are told that if they can convince a lie detector machine they are being truthful while lying, a charity will receive money. These people do not feel stressed because they are lying for an honourable reason. The machine measures stress, so it is convinced they are telling the truth.

During my life, other people have hurt me but I've convinced myself that it was my fault. I have an honourable reason for this dishonesty; if it's my fault I feel hurt, I can believe that other people are not unkind.

If other people are not unkind, I can continue to love and continue to believe I am loved.

But what I'm realising is, apart from when I was violently hurt, I didn't pay much attention to how anyone was treating me.

Even now, while seeing floods of memories through new filters, new lenses, I don't really care that much about having been hurt.

But I don't want to be hurt any more. So, I need to learn how to be more careful about who I place myself beside and how vulnerable I let myself be. And that means that while I might write about the diagnosis for now, I'm not going to talk about it. Not until I either learn *how* to speak about it, or there is far more understanding. Not until people can genuinely see that neurodiversity involves unique ways of seeing the world. Not until people can see strength and stop making assumptions about weakness, or deficit, misdiagnosis or disability. Not until people have considered that operating in groups, sharing thoughts and beliefs, attempting to be the same as one another, might not be the only, or best, way to live. And that might take much longer than my lifetime.

I know how to be silent. Silence is a parallel world—a far safer place to inhabit than hurtful conversations. As long as I can still write, I would be quite happy never to speak again.

Right now, I'm just a little bit sadder, and even lonelier.

Instead of getting upset, I distract myself by paying attention to more interesting things. Love. Writing. Cats. Reading. Drawing. Ghosts. Birds.

But I keep thinking about groups and how people mask en-masse, hiding their emotions behind shared opinions. About how groups of people have stolen entire languages and traditions from other groups in the name of some shared belief. It's heartbreaking, the lengths that groups of humans go to, have gone to, in their attempts to force other groups of humans to behave, believe and speak in exactly the same way as them. And I've spent my whole life believing that being part of a group (a community, a family, a country, a profession, friendship groups) is an ideal to aspire to.

When she diagnosed me, Dr X said, 'Instead of masking, many autistic people might simply reject what they think is expected of them. These people wander off and do their own thing.'

That made me laugh because it was the truest thing I've ever heard.

I'm not masking or hiding anything at all.

I'm gifted at wandering off. Kicking a stone along a path. Becoming invisible. Disappearing.

Cats like being talked to by humans, as long as the voice is gentle. So that's one good reason to continue to speak. Morgan likes to hear me talk. That's another.

Perhaps one day in the future, I won't speak at all any more. But for now, I'm friends with the chasing clouds and the swerving wind and the snails on the pavements.

And the cats, always the cats.

All the cats.

Sixteen Words for Loneliness

Despane– The loneliness of feeling misunderstood, unloved or unheard by someone who used to understand, love or listen.

Starn– Craving something or someone to be there but knowing it's/they're not. Wanting to bite something.

Youache– Where a specific person is missed and only their physical presence will cure the ache of missing them.

Ignornly– The kind of loneliness that other people notice, but don't mention to the person they think is lonely. Their expression shows sympathy, but also a little wariness, as if loneliness could be contagious.

Solilone– A type of melancholia experienced while gazing at a wide-skied landscape. A longing for strangeness, for the unreal or the surreal to appear.

Idealone– A hankering for an imagined scenario—where it's the idea of the situation that causes the loneliness. For example, the 'ideal' of the perfect friend sitting opposite on the sofa, laughing over wine and confessions and saying all of the right things.

Achiposs– The ache of missing out on experiencing something beautiful, because it is impossible.

Disampty– Where the immediate environment is problematic – usually in practical ways. The rubbish split all over the floor, the smoke alarm is going off, work is waiting, the clock is ticking, the umbrella's broken, it's lashing with rain and there's no one else around.

Crowdsad– Felt while around many other people. Crying while walking along streets crammed with strangers, feeling unable to speak during a burbling conversation in which others are talking loudly and not leaving any gaps.

Feartrap– when alone, overactive fears producing images of other people becoming monstrous.

Priclash– Keeping emotions or secrets private while desperately wanting to let them out.

Xiley– The loneliness of ears: usually during unexpected silence. For example, when any music player suddenly ceases to work and refuses to be fixed.

Lonmyth– the belief that no one cares / is interested, without any effort to allow people to care or show that they're interested.

Uncharm– When you realise that no matter where you go, everywhere and everyone looks almost exactly the same.

Upwrench– The rational side – loneliness needs to be felt and solitude is needed even if it's not always comfortable. Letting loneliness come, but giving it a time limit: not wallowing.

Degrag– The ache for experiences that could have been shared, but which were interrupted by tragedy.

Stone Birds

I

The storms are getting worse. A violent gale blasted through the sky all last night. I don't want to talk to anyone for a while as I've got to rethink some of my memories. Fragment them. Reassemble them. Reconsider their weight.

II

Late morning, I go outside into our garden. It's warm and the sun gleams on moist daisies. Broken twigs and pale spring leaves are scattered across damp grass.

I dissolve across the lawn, colouring myself in with greens and moisture.

Is this love for soil and earth-scent another layer, a surface-mask? It can't be. It's blood-deep. Reassembling myself with breath and movement, I walk three steps forward.

III

Crunch of white-brown sounds with my footsteps. In the gravel underneath a wooden frame which supports the tangled grapevine, there is a swarm of heavy flies.

Their thick hum vibrates the air above the ground.

The smell is solid. An organ smell.

Death.

I need to see what's lying beneath the flies. It's difficult to make myself look. To see what the flies are swarming, landing, crawling on. Feeding from.

It's three dead baby blackbirds, fallen from their nest.

One is the size of two teabags. It's made of pale skin. Its unformed wings are creased corners. Another is a little larger, darker. It has half-grown claws, tight in a coil. The third has the curls of emerging feathers. All three of them have the beginnings of beaks. Their eyes are bruises. The smudge of sight, before the eyes develop.

IV

Without speaking, I scoop up what's left of the three dead babies and wrap each of them in soft tissue. Their bodies feel oddly solid. Their skin is cold and so delicate. It's never seen daylight.

Getting a spade, I dig three small holes and bury them one at a time.

'I'm so sorry,' I whisper to each bird as I cover it with earth, 'That you never flew.'

I'm trying to pretend to myself that half of all nature is death and half is love. It's impossible to have one without the other. Everything eats everything else anyway. Everything dies. People are dying from covid and floods and fires and catastrophes all over the world. More and more every day. I am barely breathing because I'm on the verge of tears for these birds, but I should be crying for all of the people instead. I'm trying to pretend to myself that nothing bad has happened in this small garden under this small piece of sky, in this small street, on this small morning, after this violent storm, but it has.

Death is never ordinary. It can't be. It shouldn't be.

'I'm so sorry,' I whisper to the three dead birds, 'That you died before you lived.'

V

I can't speak about them all day, or the next day, or the next day. Skin. Claw. Feather.

VI

My heart feels bruised.

Occupying one of its chambers are the ghosts of the three dead birds.

The longer I can't speak about them, the heavier they're growing. Still. Solid. Blind.

266

VII

They've settled in.

The three ghost birds in my heart are small repetitions of never-growing bird-cells, splitting without expanding. They are echoes of the future-birds they never became.

They long for lightness—a trace of air felt only once, the gale that killed them.

They are the weight of a triple death—the plummet from nest to gravel. They are murderous gravity.

I still can't speak about them. I can rarely speak about the things which make me this sad.

The ghost birds are heavier than ever, today.

VIII

It's raining and I'm looking through the window at the dripping garden. The latest storm has calmed overnight. The overgrown grapevine hides an empty nest.

I'm worried about the blackbird parents. If they're returning to the nest again and again, looking for their dead chicks. If they're in the nest together now, unable to fly for grieving.

As I stare out of the rain-smeared window, the three ghost birds are stones in my heart.

They take me back through time to a stone place.

IX

I'm at my childhood home. Brick walls and concrete and stone and slate. Today I'm a sad child, fed up with everything and nothing all at the same time. Fed up with bullies hurting the poorest kids at school and fed up with the Irish reverend who's always shouting on the television and fed up with mean Margaret Thatcher and fed up with being cold and fed up with nothing being as magical as it should be. Fed up with the book I've just read, because its story ended. Fed up with maths for being made of sharp numbers which crack apart in confused crying. Fed up with the leaves being gone from the trees. Fed up with the sky for being too white and fed up with the birds for keeping their wings to themselves and fed up with my feet for always staying so firmly on the ground.

As a child the worst thing of all that I'm fed up with is that there's an invisible hole in the fireplace where the fire should be. It's dragging too many things away into it. It's taken the blue from the sky and the flowers from the hedges and the warmth from the hot water bottles. It's taken the jokes from my brothers and the laughter from my parents and the purrs from the cats. It's taken away the smells of baking and cornflakes and cinnamon, leaving the smells of damp and coal dust. It's ripped all the cardboard doors off our advent calendars and now there are no surprises. I can't explain the hole to anyone because it's making me so sad I can't speak about it. I just know the hole's there and it's pulling.

To get away from the invisible hole in the fireplace I'm playing alone outside, round the back of my childhood home. My neck is scratchy from my thick jumper. My skin is scratchy everywhere but I don't want to take any of my clothes off once they're on. The yard outside is wearing weeds as patches. Only the strongest weeds crack through the concrete.

Thistles. Prehistoric Horsetails. Nettles.

X

A narrow V of geese fly honking overhead. They're so muscular they can fly higher than this cold northern wind. They'll fly such a long way to get warmer, to eat richer foods and nest under sunshine. Their sound punches grey into my shoulder blades. If I could be a bird, I would go everywhere.

But I am stuck down here on the ground.

XI

I'm a statue-child. In my statue-world by the back door my mouth is a locked stone. In this position of claw-hands and growl-jaw, I'm a gargoyle. Tiger lips. Bird claws. With folded hands I'm an angel. I'm a dragon like this, all scales and elbow-points and hip-curves. Carved wings protect my innards as I'm hoarding a tiny flame inside my stone guts. With my head bowed I am a dead shroud-child. I am a hands-clasped gravestone child. I am brick-wall child and I am a stack-child made of concrete blocks.

Once I've become stone all the way through, I'll be completely deaf and dumb and blind. No one will make me speak. I will be as wise as three stone monkeys. I've decided not to stop being stone until something magical appears that's worth being flesh and blood for.

But it's not to be found around humans. People want everyone to be exactly the same as each other. Believe the same things, like the same things, eat the same things, wear the same things, destroy the same things, speak the same things, all while staying firmly on the ground.

XII

Be stone. Be stone. Be stone.
This is how I do it:
look at a crack in concrete.
Imagine a thousand pebbles.
Thicken the brain as a rock.
Change the heart from red into grey.
(A stone heart only beats once every thousand years. Stone locks everything in place.)
The arms in one rigid position.
Feet fused to concrete.
Ears sealed. Mouth a stone.
Closed.
In this closed world everything becomes possible:
ghosts are birds.
Children are birds.
Birds are children.
Children are ghosts.
Birds are ghosts.
All of these three things can fly when no one is looking. All of these three things can sing when no one is listening.

And as a stone child, or as a stone ghost, or as a stone bird, no matter what other people are doing, everything is solid and everything is safe and everything is locked in silence.

XIII

As a child I would often be stone until someone who knew me came right up to me and they'd shake me or clap or shout till I came back.

People who knew me would make me flesh and blood again, would make me open my eyes and voice and ears.

I wish instead of bringing me back with noise and touch they'd bring me back by singing like birds.

Singing me down from flight, so I didn't fall so suddenly and so hard.

Of course I was fine. I was fine because I'd learned what fine looked like.

Fine looked like reappearing but not being able to fly.

Fine looked like being able to easily return but not being able to sing.

Fine looked like being interested in being the same as other people, and not being the same as birds.

No one ever asked how far away I'd been.

I think the birds knew, though. They were around all the time. Storms were rarer, then.

Perhaps humans want storms to get worse because people like talking about weather.

How far away had I been?

Bird-far?

Humans don't know how far is too far. I was testing the edges of distance and never spoke about where I'd been. How high-away. How deep-away. How wide-away.

What bird-languages I'd learned to sing in.

XIV

The three ghost birds in my heart have the weight of gravity. So solid and so still.

Someone they know needs to shake them or clap or shout, to call them back to flesh and blood again.

Only I know them. But I can't even speak about them.

And I can't feed them or help them grow.

XV

Death is constantly near, for birds. Storms. Humans and their predatory pets. Human-hunger.

Imagine what would happen if all birds were capable of protecting themselves against all predators and all storms. There would be so many more of them.

If song and flight were understood as sacred, birds would be revered. They would be recognised as magical creatures.

XVI

I can't teach the three ghost birds how to fly, unless I learn how to become a bird or a ghost.

XVII

This is how I will do it:
   look at a long black feather.
   Imagine a thousand feathers.
   Lighten the brain, make it seek air.
   Feel the heart beating fast and red.
   Let it beat faster.
   (A bird's heart beats three hundred and forty-five times per minute at rest.)
   Feathers bind everything in place.
   The wings are lifted into a launching position. Feet push upwards, away from soil.
   Thump the wings down with the full force of the gravity of stones.
   Lift them again.
   Thump them down again.
   Empty the heart of sadness. Empty the heart of stone.
   Open it.
   Rise.
   Eyes open. Ears listening.
   Mouth singing, song aimed skywards.

A Loop and Three Small Stitches

I feel like a small, odd girl in the wrong time and place (it's summer in December and winter in July). I can't speak about anything important, so have decided not to speak at all. It's easy to be quiet when no one visits our house and we aren't going outside much. On Facebook and Instagram, I keep noticing conversations that say time has gone strange since the pandemic began and no one knows what month it is any more. I have stopped responding to comments, which is an easy way to be silent. From photos online, it seems that most people are only spending time with their relatives or the people they live with. Perhaps no one has friend groups any more. They have the urgent people—the home bubble, the peripheral relatives, distanced work colleagues, and solitude. The world is so loud with its pandemics and misinformation and hunger and climate emergency that no one notices if small odd girls disguised as grown women are talking or not any more.

It's a relief to be able to be quiet while I get used to the ASD diagnosis. But I also wish I could talk to someone bigger than me, someone who knows all about it. Or even just someone who knows me, from back then and back there. The places in the past where I was a child, a teenager, a young adult, a growing-older adult. I wish I knew someone else who is autistic who could help me understand what it means. Have I learned too well how to 'appear to appear'? ASD is listed as a 'disability' on job application forms. I haven't thought of myself as disabled so I tick the non-disabled box. I also tick the ASD box within the 'if you ticked yes' section. With these tick-box answers I'll appear as a contradiction before they've even seen my face.

I'm applying for more permanent jobs because I've been 'precariously employed' for a long time, but now I'm frightened about the future. Will Morgan and I be safe, or at least hopeful? Job applications are an exercise in learning how to be hopeful. Each job advert contains the possibility of a different future, though hope often seems elusive when group decisions are involved. Most employers might prefer to employ people they know, or have been guiltily exploiting for some time. Perhaps they've already decided on a particular type of person, to fill a gap. In every organisation, especially hierarchical ones, there are obvious gaps. People seem surprised when they're pointed out. Then appointments become like the process of completing jigsaws—slot in and fit. I feel sorry for the people who have to be exactly the right shape.

Online, I push myself to reach out more. Perhaps I'm wrong about groups being damaging, I've just never found the right one. As a final attempt, I join a closed Facebook group for autistic adults and in my friendly 'hello' post I write that I've very recently been diagnosed with autism and giftedness. Someone replies several times by posting four links to far-right extremism and then posting that, 'We don't use the word 'gifted' and this is why'. One of the group administrators replies to tell me, 'We have an autism first policy—you should say you're an *autistic person*. Not that you have been diagnosed with autism.'

I leave the group and try and fail not to cry for two hours.

The administrator sends me a private message to say they saw I had left, but I am eligible and welcome to join. They tell me that they educate group members about what's appropriate to say in order to protect vulnerable communities.

I reply with a message that says I don't want to hurt anyone vulnerable, but I can't join any group that tells me how to speak.

Thinking of languages being destroyed in classrooms by English-speaking teachers, I cry about all the children who were beaten by people who were part of a large group with destructive and violent beliefs. This isn't even my pain to feel, I have no right to it. But now I've started crying about loss of languages, I can't stop. Silence, when it comes from being silenced, has too many painful echoes. Echoes bounce, ricochet, multiply, collide.

The administrator sends me a message saying I can re-join the group.

I thank them for their message and tell them I can't.

Groups of humans are too difficult and dangerous.

I log out and stay logged out, retreating into silence.

Silence stops me wanting to cry. Silence is strong and safe and nothing goes wrong.

It's always gentle, this deliberate not-talking.

I don't know why I've always tried so hard, to talk.

No, I *do* know why—it's because talking-people expect all people to talk.

What I don't know, is why I'm still trying.

Since Covid began no one seems to ask, *how are you?* anymore. If they ask anything at all, it's, *are you OK?*

OK looks like a small piece of neat embroidery. A loop and three small stitches. Almost as simple as drawing a bird with just two lines.

I have no words to describe being-OK.

I have no words to describe not-being-OK.

No one is really OK or really not OK.

So many people have died. So many people are grieving. So many people are pretending that none of this is real. So many people have been stuck for months and years in locations they didn't realise they'd not be able to travel to-and-fro from.

Behind closed doors and windows, between close family members or intimate friends, perhaps OK can be untangled so that what lies beneath it can become visible.

But when close people are too far away to have intimate conversations with, and OK can't be untangled, it becomes necessary to redefine what resilience and silence really mean:

(**Resilence**– The ability to say nothing at all.)[8]

Outside, I walk around Wellington, but not as far from our home as I used to walk. Covid is now everywhere and I don't want to risk having to get a bus back because I've gone too far. Viruses love enclosed spaces. My world has shrunk to three neighbouring suburbs: Berhampore, Newtown, Island Bay. I notice the other regular solo-walking people. The man who dresses like a pirate who's stranded on the land. The gnome man with a beard and no moustache and faded green jacket who only walks in one direction. The lady in the wide-brimmed red hat. The murmuring geek guy with tangled hair.

---

8 The quietest word for loneliness. It wants to be ignored.

The lying-on-benches-groaning-with-belly-showing guy. I always see them, but they never see me because I don't want them to. These lonely people don't know it, but they need a friend who's quite like me. Like me in terms of how much I can care, how much I can see, feel, understand. But not like me right now—they need someone far more reliable. I am too lonely to help them and have no sense of permanence. For them, I would be at best a disappointing friend and at worst, an abandoning or damaging one.

But would that be still better than having no friends at all? They can't see me because I've made myself completely invisible to everyone, today. They don't want anything from me and I don't want anything from them.

This is what loneliness really is when it's gone beyond itself, to its darkest place. An impotent binding. I am tied in, and in tying myself in, others are shut out. Like a spell that ties threads around a poppet, to stop someone harming themselves or others.

But why are so many other people also walking past these lonely people, without seeming to even see them? These walking people look far more permanent than me—they belong and will always live here. They walk with purpose, reliably expected to return to their homes and jobs and social locations. But their averted gaze and rapid movement makes me feel that humans don't know how to live well together, even though so many of us live right beside one another. Why don't people care more than they seem to, or at least speak about how much they care, more often?

Is there some kind of an agreement between people that I might have missed? About not saying what we feel, or not when we first meet each other. Acquaintances like to make small talk or say hello and walk away. I'm not very good at the small talk or walking away bit, because I want to talk about and listen to interesting things. I start caring for people as soon as they tell me something personal, no matter how small. Is the way I care dangerous for them? That's not going to change, because I don't want it to. I want to care.

Maybe humans don't care about each other until they feel deeply known. Why not care about each other before we know each other? Why not care about everyone who hasn't yet proved to us that we shouldn't? Or is this dangerous?

It's so easy to be bound and invisible. Just think of stone. Think of being closed.

My eyes have a lonely-filter at the moment. I am too homesick. I miss too much, even people and places I never deeply knew. I can tell there's a lonely-filter because I'm only noticing the broken things. I'm noticing tiny signs of loneliness all around me. A stained window with a teddy bear in it. An upstairs window with an A4 piece of paper showing the desperate word 'hello' in faded pen. A broken wine bottle scattered across the pavement. Blocks of flats with mouldy walls. Rusted tin roofs. The concrete beneath my feet feels thin. I look up at the posts that support tangled electricity wires and light bulbs, wondering if they'll fall in an earthquake. If the lights will all go out, like eyes closing.

If the lights all go out, what will the future become? I imagine everyone in all the houses in all the streets in all the cities of the world quietly singing to themselves in the dark. No news. No social media. No long-distance voices.

I am learning to speak into the gaps made by things which have gone.

We don't need as many humans around us as we think.

Just one or two, perhaps a few occasionally. The ones who care. There are so many who don't.

Look away.

Gone.

If the lights all go out, what will the future become?

Sometimes, it's necessary to enlist the help of birds.

All the birds will hear our lonely singing and invent brighter, happier, songs.

If the lights all go out, what will the future become?

Every dawn, the birds sing choruses of hope.

They open the world with light by singing the sun out of the ocean, up, up, up, into the sky.

If all the lights go on, what will the future become?

Eighteen Words for Loneliness

Despane– The loneliness of feeling misunderstood, unloved or unheard by someone who used to understand, love or listen.

Starn– Craving something or someone to be there but knowing it's/ they're not. Wanting to bite something.

Youache– Where a specific person is missed and only their physical presence will cure the ache of missing them.

Ignornly– The kind of loneliness that other people notice, but don't mention to the person they think is lonely. Their expression shows sympathy, but also a little wariness, as if loneliness could be contagious.

Solilone– A type of melancholia experienced while gazing at a wide-skied landscape. A longing for strangeness, for the unreal or the surreal to appear.

Idealone– A hankering for an imagined scenario—where it's the idea of the situation that causes the loneliness. For example, the 'ideal' of the perfect friend sitting opposite on the sofa, laughing over wine and confessions and saying all of the right things.

Achiposs– The ache of missing out on experiencing something beautiful, because it is impossible.

Disampty– Where the immediate environment is problematic – usually in practical ways. The rubbish split all over the floor, the smoke alarm is going off, work is waiting, the clock is ticking, the umbrella's broken, it's lashing with rain and there's no one else around.

Crowdsad– Felt while around many other people. Crying while walking along streets crammed with strangers, feeling unable to speak during a burbling conversation in which others are talking loudly and not leaving any gaps.

Feartrap– when alone, overactive fears producing images of other people becoming monstrous.

Priclash– Keeping emotions or secrets private while desperately wanting to let them out.

Xiley– The loneliness of ears: usually during unexpected silence. For example, when any music player suddenly ceases to work and refuses to be fixed.

Lonmyth– the belief that no one cares / is interested, without any effort to allow people to care or show that they're interested.

Uncharm– When you realise that no matter where you go, everywhere and everyone looks almost exactly the same.

Upwrench– The rational side – loneliness needs to be felt and solitude is needed even if it's not always comfortable. Letting loneliness come, but giving it a time limit: not wallowing.

Degrag– The ache for experiences that could have been shared, but which were interrupted by tragedy.

Resilence– The ability to say nothing at all.

Yorch– The final kick just before you're about to be reunited with a person/people who you've missed.

Light

In about five months from now, when Morgan is diagnosed with autism too, my eyes will change their filter.

We'll be sitting side-by-side at the table in front of her computer screen. She'll turn to me with shining eyes. She'll say, 'See—we're exactly the same.'

I'll grip her hand, watching her carefully to check she's all right.

She will be all right, because she's already sure of who she is.

'We're bonobos, not chimps,' she'll grin at me. 'Didn't I say?'

She'll shut the computer down and we'll stand up and hug and she'll say, 'Let's celebrate tonight.' She'll have a slightly sore hip from climbing a steep hill with me the day before. I'll be the one who goes outside to buy us a bottle of bubbles.

While I'm walking along the path that leads down to Island Bay and the supermarket, I'll be thinking about what Morgan's feeling at home. I'll feel her walking around the rooms, sitting down in the comfy chair that looks out at the garden. I'll feel her breathe out as her eyes soak in many shades of green. Her emotions echo; a lack of surprise, a feeling of certainty.

Beside her in our home, I'll invisibly put my hand on her shoulder.

Beside me on the path, she'll invisibly take my hand.

I'll stop walking. I'll look upwards through tall trees and examine the bright-clouded sky. I'll have become aware with a gasp that I have a new feeling. All around me, colours will become a little brighter. The wind will move the grass to whispers and the textures of dry pine needles across the path will be highlighted by shadows.

I'll still feel her hand in mine. We used to touch like this from opposite sides of the world.

I'll test the new feeling, not quite trusting it. I'll flurry at it. Retreat from it. Breathe into it. Breathe it out to see if it leaves me quickly.

I'll notice that the new feeling is tentative, but it's not flitting away—

I don't feel quite so lonely. It's still there, but lighter, gentler.

This feeling will change how I'm seeing everything as I turn off the path and walk along the pavements of Island Bay towards the supermarket.

My eyes will have a together-filter and I'll only notice things which are linked together. A window with a newly washed teddy bear in it for children to wave at. An upstairs window with an A4 piece of paper showing the word 'hello!' in bright purple pen. A celebratory wine bottle scattered across the pavement—evidence of a party. Ivy stems finding rootholds in the cracks of walls, young leaves embracing older ones as if they have empathy. Waterproof tin roofs, waiting to give sound to welcome rain. The ground beneath my feet will feel steady. A footfall, held up. The concrete, pressed down.

Inside my chest I'll feel an opening instead of a closing. I won't know what it is but I'll notice the new feeling again—

I don't feel quite so lonely.

I'll look up at the tangled electricity wires and believe that electricity—the way it chases all along these wires from one home to another and from one person to another—is made of some kind of magic.

The Empathy of Leaves

Tonight, I'm outside in our neighbour's tree which is so big I'm convinced its roots have vaults. I'm perched on a branch between a pair of roosting kererū who don't know I'm here. I feel the coldness of the air between their plump bodies as an embrace.

All around me the leaves whisper to each other. They're murmuring about roots and fire and ice and stones and clouds and miraculous water and the height birds can fly to and the tunnels huhu grubs make in beautifully decaying wood...

'Even worms need something solid to hold onto,' say the leaves. 'And when they find it, they writhe through it.'

I tell the leaves, 'Thank goodness I've got Morgan. I need something to hold onto too.'

Their murmurs rise like laughter and spread from leaf veins into branches. 'We all do!' The leaves quieten as they reply, 'We know what you're thinking.'

'Do you?' I hadn't realised that leaves are able to read the minds of humans. But it's possible. Trees communicate with each other though their roots. They also communicate with each other through air, using scents. Whenever I walk home along Adelaide Road at night-time, I raise my hand to touch my fingers to the hanging leaves of all the trees. I can tell when they want it to rain and when they're in shock about one of their own, falling.

I know all the trees around here. Perhaps they know me too.

The leaves speak quietly. 'You dreamed you were a ghost, last night. Your dream fell downwards and thudded all through the soil.'

The dream has made me sad all day and I've been trying not to think about it, but now I have to. My empty body was in the same room in Scotland my dad died in. Sitting at the table with its eyes closed. As a ghost, I stood beside it, watching. Living people moved through me, making arrangements for my body to leave the room. And all the while I looked and looked and looked at my body. I wanted to slip into it again but there was no way back in. It was too solid.

My body was a home I couldn't go back to.

My dad wasn't there either. In the dream I was there because I was looking for him, but I found myself instead, dead.

The leaves are still murmuring a half-missed conversation. '... wandering away and wandering back again.'

I touch a few leaf tips with my finger. 'You're clever and beautiful. Your thin stems. Your layers and delicate edges. These green tones. Photosynthesis. Does it feel—'

The leaves say, 'Part of you is like a child. Part of your father was also like a child.'

'The few people I love most, are. They still draw. Paint. Read. Write stories. Talk about love. Play musical instruments. See all kinds of things when they look into fires and rivers and oceans and clouds.'

'You're so often sad,' say the leaves. 'Even though you see intense beauty everywhere.'

I tell them the truth. 'I'm sad because my dad is a ghost and I don't know where he is. And I'm stuck here on the ground, unable to travel back across the world, or back through time, to find him.'

The leaves whisper-laugh. 'Time's simultaneous, not linear.'

I frown. 'Are you sure?'

Another whisper-laugh. 'You're gifted at wandering away and wandering back again. So wander off. Go and find him.'

The Symbols of Birds and Ghosts

While he was dying, my dad drew the same shape over and over again in a small sketchbook. I asked him what the drawing was. He said he was trying to draw the perfect symbol and told me the heart shape within his symbol represented love. He said more than this and gave the symbol a particular name, *symbol perfecta* or *perfecto* or *perfecti*? He struggled to name it—to find the right words. There was an additional vowel sound somewhere, but because his language was jumbled, my memory has covered this conversation in clouds.

My dad's small sketchbook is now hidden in my desk drawer. I've only looked at it once since he died—there are too many blank pages at the end. But F, my friend who writes to me on Messenger, recently told me about a strange dream he'd had about a symbol drawn on the roof so helicopters could land. Now I keep thinking about symbols. I can ignore the blank pages this time. I've cried enough about them.

I open the drawer and remove my dad's cloth-covered sketchbook. Sitting on the sofa, I turn the pages tenderly. I'm trying to preserve whatever's left of his touch. Fingerprints, skin cells. The sketchbook contains drawings in felt-tip pens and pastels. There are drawings of bright patterns, green tunnels and labyrinths. There's also a drawing of a bird that he and I invented together by taking turns to draw one line at a time, not speaking. The bird is brightly coloured, hunch-shouldered, multi-feathered. A parrot with the curved bill of a toucan.

On a page about half-way through the book he's drawn a symbol I don't recognise—and written words beneath it: *cho ku rei*. I look online and find it's a Reiki symbol. Reiki is a Japanese method of spiritual healing my dad learned and practiced. This symbol is used to increase or decrease power, depending on the direction it's drawn. A few pages later, there's another Reiki symbol and *sei he ki*. Online, there are two possible meanings and because he's drawn green lines and roots beneath different shades of blue, I know he chose the meaning: 'the earth and sky meet'. There are more pages, mainly patterns, some of them brightly coloured, others in more subdued tones. He's written a phrase from a Dylan Thomas poem[9] in red and orange pastels: *Rage, Rage, against the dying of the light.* And beneath these bright words, he's written in pencil, *do not go gentle into that good night.*

There's a folded square of kitchen towel placed over this page to protect the unfixed colours. Pastel drawings are fixed by spraying the page with hairspray when the picture is complete. The presence of the kitchen towel shows he considered this page unfinished.

Unfixed *do not go* unfinished *night.*

Unfinished *rage.*

Unfixed *dying light.*

Gentle is gone.

I whisper to no one, 'This is still too hard.'

Morgan's been writing for a while in the other room. She comes in to get the lead for her laptop and asks how I'm doing.

I reply, 'I'm looking at my dad's last sketchbook.'

She asks, 'And are you all right?'

In the doorway behind her, something moves in the air. A movement of lines, visible, invisible. Staring without blinking, I say, 'I'm not quite sure what I'm seeing.'

Morgan turns to look. She says, 'It's a daddy longlegs, caught on a cobweb that's come down from the ceiling. Poor thing.'

Now I know what it is, I can see it. It's a winged creature with long legs, pulling on a long and tangled web-thread. Leaving the sofa, I grab the end of the thread and let the insect gently pull me towards the light shining through the open back door.

It moves in slow circles above my head, making a tiny whirring sound. Morgan is mesmerised, watching.

She calls, 'That's the sweetest thing I've seen for a long time. It's leading you outside.'

For a moment I feel like a small girl made of spray-paint; Banksy's famous graffiti of the little girl with a balloon on a string. Did my dad ever see that picture? I'm not sure if we ever talked about Banksy. We should have talked about Banksy.

Out in the garden, I carefully untangle the insect's frail legs from sticky threads.

---

9   Dylan Thomas, *Do not go gentle into that good night.*

It flies off as if nothing bad has ever happened to it.

It's quiet, today. Sometimes the neighbours are all out at the same time, but today it's just me and the garden birds who are chattering to each other across the fences.

Morgan goes back into the other room.

I wash web threads from my fingertips before I return to my dad's sketchbook.

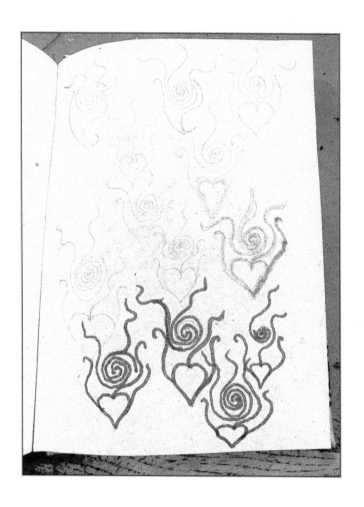

Alan Richards's final sketchbook

I try to remember what he'd called his perfect symbol. Perhaps the name doesn't matter. What matters is that the symbol changed slightly each time he drew it. At first there's a v shape and swirling lines in pencil. These are repeated until the v evolves into the shape of a love heart beneath a spiral. There are signs of weakness in the wavering pencil lines. The final symbols are more definite, the spiral is confident, the flowing lines more decisive, colours are chosen. Blue, then grey, then on the next page, it becomes purple.

The love hearts fatten. Full of purple love. Heavy with it?

What does the spiral symbolise? One line meets another and another, in a careful series of coils and curves. A double spiral, with a gap in the centre. What does a whirlpool, a spring, a vortex, or a coil mean? With more online searches I find images of double spirals described as 'hinged' spirals, but though the central part is similar, the additional flowing lines and the love heart in my dad's drawing make it different. My memory is accurate in some respects; this was a symbol he was inventing while he was dying.

I wonder if any pages in my dad's sketchbook are written in invisible ink and contain hidden messages, secret code. This is how conspiracy theories and fictions begin to form.

But there is no secret code. All meanings belonged to my dad and he's now unaskable. All I can do is make a note of what I see—

My dad's perfect symbol is a full heart beneath a swirling multi-directional spiral. The heart is weighted to occupy the ground while some of its emotions drift up into the air. A double spiral is airborne. The spiral represents something which flies along a curved route in order to meet itself, reverse its direction and fly away.

Air, spirit, cloud. Bird, ghost, love.

This sketchbook and his camera are the only things I have here, that he touched. Checking my wrists for traces of sticky cobweb, I clasp the sketchbook over my heart.

When I was little I was terrified of daddy longlegs. My dad used to come and catch them in the bedroom I shared with my little brother. I was so terrified of them I either screamed or froze. He'd catch them and put them outside. I was annoyed with myself for being frightened and decided to draw them from memory. I'd draw one tiny part of the insect at a time. Angular legs, sectioned bodies. Corners, where the legs bent in sinister angles. I had pure fear, when sitting back and looking at the whole drawing. Pure fear was what I needed. It meant the drawing was successful. I'd cover the drawing with a piece of paper, look at it for one second, then cover it again. Then two seconds and cover it again. Three seconds. And so on.

Eventually I could sleep in the same room as a daddy longlegs without screaming or freezing because I trained myself not to fear them by drawing them over and over again.

What did my dad's repetitive drawing of this symbol do for him while he was dying? Did drawing that full heart and those spirals give him fear or comfort?

I'm getting lost in other fears. It's a bad anniversary—this is the time of year he became suddenly sick and died. The fear is that this grief will never go away, a sense of something wrong within my body, a raw ache-hole that expands. I could draw a picture or symbol of the hole, cover it over and look at it again, but it wouldn't help. The drawing couldn't show this fear of speaking and not being able to speak for crying. The fear of crying and not being able to stop.

The fear of uncontrollable thoughts. I keep thinking of all the things he didn't do, as well as all the things he did.

I'm afraid of all the things I don't know as well as all the things I do know.

I'm afraid of not being able to control torturous thoughts—my thoughts of all the things he might have done if he hadn't died.

It's almost unbearable, at the time of this bad anniversary, that there are no new memories.

On Facebook my aunt sends me a photograph of a handwritten letter my dad wrote when he was nine years old.

She writes that she misses him too. She writes that *he so loved birds.*

The shadow of her phone falls over the image. I leave the screen-letter, go and cry, come back and look at the screen-letter again.

The letter has a Winchester address printed in the top right corner. The stamped-on date is the 28th of January 1956. It's written over in pen to make it clearer.

A third of the way down the handwritten letter the ink runs out and is replaced.

The letter is not addressed to anyone:

I am going to be a Bird Naturalist when I grow up.
Today I have seen—
4 Blackbirds, 1 coal tit, 3 Great Tits, 5 Bluetits, 9 Starlings, 4
Thrushes (Mistle and Song) and 9 Rooks.
Where seen:— Blackbirds, tree in our garden. Thrushes ' ' ' ' Tits,
(Coal, Blue and Great) on Fat in our garden. Starlings } on floor
in our garden. Rooks in air above our garden.
WRITTEN BY
Alan Richards

The little boy who wrote this letter to no one had a violent father. This nine-year-old version of my dad wanted something so badly which was fully realised just before he died, after many years of hard work. This little boy who wrote lists of birds might have been autistic and struggling, but no one understood. Was he lonely? I've been trying to think logical thoughts about symbols but seeing this letter and not being able to touch it, or hug this child-version of my dad, hurts.

Tonight, my thoughts are whirring insects around my head.
  My heart collapses through a dad-sized hole.
  I am small, the size of a daughter.
  Morgan is asleep in bed. I'm outside in the garden and there are clouds in the night sky. Orion is upside down and a wing-shaped cloud passes across his head and shoulders. Weightless.
  Up there in mirrored stars, no harm is done. Everything is light.
  But what is the weight of a daughter's heart?
  It is heavy and full. It lies on the earth beside my feet, attached to my body with tangled silk threads.
  I want to be here, but I am almost not-here.
  I want to be there, but I am almost not-there.

He will never come to me here in New Zealand. Like me, he doesn't belong here.
  And I am not loud enough to call him in any way he can hear me.
  The world turns over and under itself.
  The dead are busy elsewhere.
  They have no sense of time, or not in the way that the living do.

The dead exist across this moment and this one and this one.
These moments are not linear, they are simultaneous.
He can only be found in the places he called home.

I close my eyes and crouch. I am covered in a thousand feathers. I thump my wings down with the full force of the gravity of stones. Lift them again. Thump them down again. Open the heart.

Rise.

Eyes open. Ears listening for echoes of birdsong.

Wings whirr.

Daylight.

The nine-year-old version of my father is watching birds in a garden in Winchester.

I circle through the air as he sits under a tree writing in his notebook. Three small blackbirds flutter away from somewhere beneath me, as if they're learning to fly.

As a starling, I land beside him in the grass.

I chirrup into his ear that I know his father is violent and his mother is silent and then I whistle at him to tell him he's loved by a wife and four grown-up children and their lovers and his eldest grand-daughter who loved him and his youngest grand-daughter who was born around a month after he died, and lots of other people he taught and met and played music with and showed forests and woods and trees and leaves to, other people he showed gannets and starlings and eagles and cormorants and oystercatchers to, and I sing to him that he's seen more birds than are on any list.

My boy-dad examines me with shining eyes. He writes in his notebook:

There is a giant talking Starling in my garden.

He turns and hugs me, small arms holding me tight. I pick him up on my back and fly north with him, carrying him to the place where he will volunteer when he's retired.

He's sleepy when we arrive at the shed with a tin roof where my dad's ghost is sitting at a trestle table, counting the seabirds he's seen that day:

8 Ghost-Kittiwakes,
3 Phantom-Cormorants,
1 Spirit-Guillemot,
4 Ghoul-Gannets...

Dropping my boy-dad gently onto a wooden seat, my heart pulls at me. Far away, Morgan stirs in her sleep. I feel her settle again. 'Soon,' I whisper to her, 'I promise. I'll come home, soon.'

My boy-dad examines my ghost-dad's notebook. Seeing lists of birds, moths, numbers, locations, he sighs with contentment. He leans against my ghost-dad, who puts his hand on my boy-dad's shoulder.

I leave them together in the shed, shutting the door behind me. For a long while, their high and low voices murmur excitedly.

Outside, pale sunlight glistens on the sea and clouds are chased by high currents of wind. In this field on top of the cliffs, long grass moves in circles. My limbs ache from flying and my hands are transparent.

My heart beats in a distant place. Return, return. Return, return. Return, return.

I have been gone too long, again.

Can I leave them here now and trust that they're safe and happy?

I wait for a while, feeling the ice in the wind. Becoming part of the ice in the wind. Is it possible to be certain of anything in this in-between place?

The sound of footfall from inside the shed. I turn around as the shed door opens. My ghost-dad and boy-dad walk hand-in-hand towards the cliffs. They walk along the cliff edge for a while, watching gannets plunge into the waves. They turn and face the sky.

Ghost-dad spreads his arms wide.

Boy-dad spreads his.

My transparent hands cover my mouth.

They both run to the very edge of the cliff and keep running as the ground falls away and they vanish.

Tears flow over my fingertips. I watch them without blinking.

Two albatrosses, one large and one small, wheel through the clouds.

They draw invisible lines in the sky.
They belong here, they've always belonged here.
Exactly like this.

My dad's perfect symbol is a full heart beneath a swirling multi-directional spiral. The heart is weighted to occupy the ground while some of its emotions drift up into the air. A double spiral is airborne. The spiral represents something which flies along a curved route in order to meet itself, reverse its direction and fly away.

Air, spirit, cloud. Bird, ghost, love.

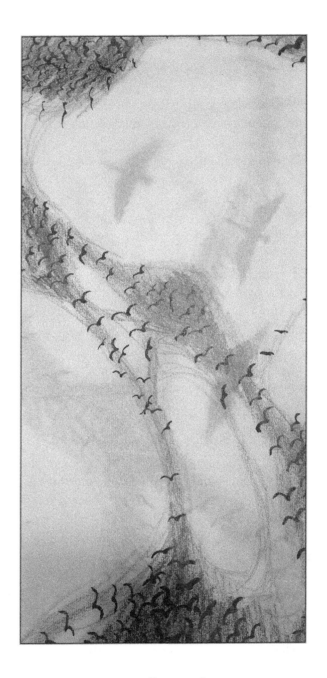

Travelling Light

Nineteen Words for Loneliness

Despane– The loneliness of feeling misunderstood, unloved or unheard by someone who used to understand, love or listen.

Starn– Craving something or someone to be there but knowing it's/ they're not. Wanting to bite something.

Youache– Where a specific person is missed and only their physical presence will cure the ache of missing them.

Ignornly– The kind of loneliness that other people notice, but don't mention to the person they think is lonely. Their expression shows sympathy, but also a little wariness, as if loneliness could be contagious.

Solilone– A type of melancholia experienced while gazing at a wide-skied landscape. A longing for strangeness, for the unreal or the surreal to appear.

Idealone– A hankering for an imagined scenario—where it's the idea of the situation that causes the loneliness. For example, the 'ideal' of the perfect friend sitting opposite on the sofa, laughing over wine and confessions and saying all of the right things.

Achiposs– The ache of missing out on experiencing something beautiful, because it is impossible.

Disampty– Where the immediate environment is problematic – usually in practical ways. The rubbish split all over the floor, the smoke alarm is going off, work is waiting, the clock is ticking, the umbrella's broken, it's lashing with rain and there's no one else around.

Crowdsad– Felt while around many other people. Crying while walking along streets crammed with strangers, feeling unable to speak during a burbling conversation in which others are talking loudly and not leaving any gaps.

Feartrap– when alone, overactive fears producing images of other people becoming monstrous.

Priclash– Keeping emotions or secrets private while desperately wanting to let them out.

Xiley– The loneliness of ears: usually during unexpected silence. For example, when any music player suddenly ceases to work and refuses to be fixed.

Lonmyth– the belief that no one cares / is interested, without any effort to allow people to care or show that they're interested.

Uncharm– When you realise that no matter where you go, everywhere and everyone looks almost exactly the same.

Upwrench– The rational side – loneliness needs to be felt and solitude is needed even if it's not always comfortable. Letting loneliness come, but giving it a time limit: not wallowing.

Degrag– The ache for experiences that could have been shared, but which were interrupted by tragedy.

Resilence– The ability to say nothing at all.

Yorch– The final kick just before you're about to be reunited with a person/people who you've missed.

Relonate– The realisation that persistent loneliness enables you to connect deeply with all kinds of creatures.

Listen More Closely to the Birds

In our garden in Wellington,
a nest; expanding through thickening rose leaves
inside the eggs: the early stages of dark feathers, the edge of a claw.
Half-nightmare, half-beak, made of hunger.
Open, close. Open, close.

> *The best nest must:*
> *be out of reach of cats,*
> *be made from strong materials,*
> *not have holes*
> *never sway during gales.*
> *The best nest must:*
> *be out of reach of humans.*

> *If a human enters your nest, death visits.*

In these urban back gardens
thin fences separate one set of humans from another.

> *Don't get too close.*

Don't look for an invisible bird on invisible eggs.
Don't clap at the neighbour's cat, stalking something invisible.
Don't hold an empty nest, don't cradle it.
Don't overthink the transformation of house into home.

> *Beak grips twig, pincer-tight*
> *don't touch the tongue to*
> *bad luck.*

I keep wondering if right now the world seems
unpredictable and dangerous to birds as well.
What do the birds say to each other up there in the clouds—

watch out, don't breathe whatever it is they're breathing.
Have humans gone from the sky
or are they pretending?

the sky is empty of aeroplanes
and full of chattering squawking shrieking birds.
This is where we are.

This is where we are

Sometimes there's this sound

learning to scream.

or another sound; owls at night-time.
Phone-images of miniature ghouls, faceless
flocks of mesh wings, elastic necks—
thin, breakable.

Tonight the wind and my mum call me on Skype.
She's at home in Scotland,
her bathed hair shines henna-orange.
Behind her face, bird-silhouette stickers on window panes.

'You should have visited ages ago. And you're still not here. Bloody
corvid.'
Covid sounds
    oddly pixelated.

Over her shoulder
the wind swirls around her stone house.
Roof slates slide, skitter, crash.

    derelict hours

Derelict owls
separated by gales.

Search for eyes behind the screen in my mum's glasses.
Disappear into that blur around the windows.

I imagine my dad appearing faintly—
a ghost-man,
flying in as a bird, tapping his beak on the screen in bird-tap-code,
telling me he only pretended to die.

That is a lie
a lie
a lie.

My mum's voice:
    'I've been making knitted leaves.
    a vine to bind them all together.
    Keeping all the doors open
    to let the house breathe.'

Eyes glinting, hugging the screen a wing-goodbye
as un-named crows we hang up.
Click, close.

Once upon a time a blackbird flew
straight into the jaws of a tabby cat.
Dead in a bite.

All over the world there are superstitions about death
and birds flying into houses.

Humans invent
their own bad luck.

Here in New Zealand pīwakawaka announce death
by flying in through open doors and windows.

Over there in Scotland, any bird who dies indoors predicts death-
in-the-house.
I boarded a plane three months after my dad died.

Flying off chasing love.
Flitting across this whole world chasing survival.

This is where we are.

We don't need as many humans around us as we think.
Just one or two, perhaps a few occasionally. The ones who care.
There are so many who don't.
Look away.
Gone.

> *This is where we are.*
> *Listen for us, we've got languages of hope and joy!*

Morgan's voice,
  ' sweetheart?'
My reply,

    '   a tangle head. It'll pass.'
hand squeeze

an agreement
a whisper,
'Thank you, for you.'

   —I'm in three places:
One part of me is here in New Zealand with Morgan,
the person I love most in the whole world.
Another part is in Scotland giving my mum a feathered crow-hug.
Another part has time-travelled away through open doors and
windows

> *We break our necks on your glass skies.*

no-past   no-present
every story I have ever told is being re-written in three ways:
by diagnosis, by love, by grief

the future is suspended in air.

Advice to all lonely humans:

keep listening for unfamiliar noises.
The future has a strange-sounding voice.
You'll know it when you hear it, calling.

Be beside someone who uses languages you understand.
Listen closely to everything that flies or swims or grows right
beside you.
Be as quiet or as loud as your opening-closing heart demands.

I am learning to speak in the language of birds and ghosts.

Open, close.

Open, close.

Open, close.

Acknowledgements

With thanks to the following wonderful humans: Kingsley Baird, Jonathan Board, Diane Comer, Thom Conroy, Jess Chubb, Lynley Edmeades, Gigi Fenster, Naomi Foyle, Gill Greer, Rebecca Holden, Robert Hurley, Natasha Lampard, Rachael Lowe, Lucy Luck, Lynn Michell, Melody Nixon, Bek Pickard, Anne Richards, Jonathan Ruppin, Lisa Samuels, Emma Sweeney, Sam Trubridge, Carrie Ziemke-Dickens.

With thanks to the following wonderful cats: Boy, Danu, Fliss, Fudge, Gwennie, Saffy and Toto.

And with all my heart, thank you for you, Morgan.

'Ghosts Have No Feet' was first published in Landfall 244, NZ, November 2022.

'The Ghost in the Room' was first published in Headland Literary Journal, NZ, 2022.

'To Butterfly a Ghost' and 'Stop Being Thistledown' were first published in The Saltbush Review, Issue 2, Australia, 2022.

'Beauty, Sleeping' was first published in On Repair: Performance Research 26:4. (Routledge Journals) 2022.

'The Language of Birds and Ghosts' was first published in Fresh Ink Anthology, Cloud Ink Press, NZ, 2021.

'Secrets of a Stitchbird' was first published in Ambit Magazine 245, UK, 2021.

A version of 'After-Humans' was first published in Wingless Dreamer, Literary Magazine, UK, 2021.

A few of the drawings have been published in: Fresh Ink Anthology,

NZ. Beyond Words Literary and Arts Magazine, Germany. Deluge Literary and Arts Magazine, USA, 2020-21.

'Nineteen Words for Loneliness' was adapted from my list of fifteen words for loneliness, first published in my third novel, *City of Circles*, Sceptre, 2017.

CPSIA information can be obtained
at www.ICGtesting.com
Printed in the USA
BVHW052300010223
657634BV00012B/230